EVIDENCE BASED MEDICINE IN

General Practice

EVIDENCE-BASED MEDICINE
—— *in* ——
General Practice

Dermot P.B. McGovern
MB BS, MRCP
Research Fellow, Gastroenterology Department,
University of Oxford, UK

William S.M. Summerskill
AB, MB BS, MSc
(Evidence Based Health Care), DRCOG,
DCH, DFFP, MRCGP
General Practitioner, Saintbridge Surgery
Gloucester, UK

Roland M. Valori
MB BS, MSc
(Evidence Based Healthcare), MD, FRCP
Consultant Gastroenterologist,
Gloucestershire Royal Hospital, Gloucester, UK

Marcel Levi
MD, PhD
Chairman, Department of Medicine,
Academic Medical Centre,
University of Amsterdam, The Netherlands

Richard J. McManus
MSc, MB BS, MRCP
General Practitioner and Clinical Research Fellow,
University of Birmingham, UK

Published in a modified form for hospital doctors as Key Topics in Evidence-Based Medicine by D.P.B. McGovern, W.S.M. Summerskill, R.M. Valori, and M. Levi. Published by BIOS Scientific Publishers in 2001

First published 2001

A CIP catalogue record for this book is available from the British Library.

ISBN 1 85996 282 3

BIOS Scientific Publishers Ltd
9 Newtec Place, Magdalen Road, Oxford OX4 1RE, UK
Tel. +44 (0)1865 726286. Fax +44 (0)1865 246823
World Wide Web home page: http://www.bios.co.uk/

Important Note from the Publisher
The information contained within this book was obtained by BIOS Scientific Publishers Ltd from sources believed by us to be reliable. However, while every effort has been made to ensure its accuracy, no responsibility for loss or injury whatsoever occasioned to any person acting or refraining from action as a result of information contained herein can be accepted by the authors or publishers.

The reader should remember that medicine is a constantly evolving science and while the authors and publishers have ensured that all dosages, applications and practices are based on current indications, there may be specific practices which differ between communities. You should always follow the guidelines laid down by the manufacturers of specific products and the relevant authorities in the country in which you are practising.

Production Editor: Andrea Bosher
Typeset by Jayvee Computer Services, Trivandrum, India
Printed by T.J. International, Padstow, UK

CONTENTS

Application

Index

ABBREVIATIONS

A&E	Accident and Emergency
AAA	abdominal aortic aneurysm
AF	atrial fibrillation
AMI	acute myocardial infarction
ARI	absolute risk increase
ARIF	Aggressive Research Intelligence Facility
ARR	absolute risk reduction
CBT	cognitive behaviour therapy
CER	controlled event rate
CHD	coronary heart disease
CHImp/CHI	Commission for Health Improvement
CI	confidence interval
CINAHL	Cumulative Index to Nursing & Allied Health
CPGs	clinical practice guidelines
DALYs	disability-adjusted life-year
EBM	evidence-based medicine
EER	experimental event rate
EPOC	Effective Practice and Organisation of Care
GPRD	General Practice Research Database
HeaLYs	healthy life-years
HIS	Health Interview Survey
HRQL	health-related quality of life
HTA	Health Technology Assessment (programme)
IHD	ischaemic heart disease
ITT	intention to treat
MeSH	Medical Sub Headings
NELH	National Electronic Library
NHS CRP	NHS Centre for Reviews and Dissemination
NKA	National Institute for Clinical Excellence
NNH	number(s) needed to harm
NNS	number(s) needed to screen
NNT	number(s) needed to treat
NSF	National Service Framework
OCP	oral contraceptive pill
PEER	patients expected event rate
QALYs	quality-adjusted life years
RCT	randomized controlled trial
RR	relative risk
RRR	relative risk reduction
RS	rating scales
SG	standard gamble
SIGLE	Systems for information on Grey Literature in Europe
SIGN	Scottish Intercollegiate Guidelines Network

TTO	time trade-off
TURP	transurethral resection of the prostate
VOD	veno-occlusive disease
YHL	years of healthy life
YHLL	years of healthy life lost

Names of Medical Substances

In accordance with directive 92/27/EEC, this book adheres to the following guidelines on naming of medicinal substances (rINN, Recommended International Non-proprietary Name; BAN, British Approved Name).

List 1 – Both names to appear

UK Name	rINN
[1]adrenaline	epinephrine
amethocaine	tetracaine
bendrofluazide	bendroflumethiazide
benzhexol	trihexyphenidyl
chlorpheniramine	chlorphenamine
dicyclomine	dicycloverine
dothiepin	dosulepin
eformoterol	formoterol
flurandrenolone	fludroxycortide
frusemide	furosemide
hydroxyurea	hydroxycarbamide
lignocaine	lidocaine
methotrimeprazine	levomepromazine
methylene blue	methylthioninium chloride
mitozantrone	mitoxantrone
mustine	chlormethine
nicoumalone	acenocoumarol
[1]noradrenaline	norepinephrine
oxypentifylline	pentoxifylline
procaine penicillin	procaine benzylpenicillin
salcatonin	calcitonin (salmon)
thymoxamine	moxisylyte
thyroxine sodium	levothyroxine sodium
trimeprazine	alimemazine

List 2 – rINN to appear exclusively

Former BAN	rINN/new BAN
amoxycillin	amoxicillin
amphetamine	amfetamine
amylobarbitone	amobarbital
amylobarbitone sodium	amobarbital sodium
beclomethasone	beclometasone
benorylate	benorilate
busulphan	busulfan
butobarbitone	butobarbital
carticaine	articane
cephalexin	cefalexin
cephamandole nafate	cefamandole nafate
cephazolin	cefazolin
cephradine	cefradine
chloral betaine	cloral betaine
chlorbutol	chlorobutanol
chlormethiazole	clomethiazole
chlorathalidone	chlortalidone
cholecalciferol	colecalciferol
cholestyramine	colestyramine
clomiphene	clomifene
colistin sulphomethate sodium	colistimethate sodium
corticotrophin	corticotropin
cysteamine	mercaptamine
danthron	dantron
desoxymethasone	desoximetasone
dexamphetamine	dexamfetamine
dibromopropamidine	dibrompropamidine
dienoestrol	dienestrol
dimethicone(s)	dimeticone
dimethyl sulphoxide	dimethyl sulfoxide
doxycycline hydrochloride (hemihydrate hemiethanolate)	doxycycline hyclate
ethancrynic acid	etacrynic acid
ethamsylate	etamsylate
ethinyloestradiol	ethinylestradiol
ethynodiol	etynodiol
flumethasone	flumetasone
flupenthixol	flupentixol
gestronol	gestonorone
guaiphenesin	guaifenesin

[1] In common with the BP, precedence will continue to be given to the terms adrenaline and noradrenaline.

hexachlorophane	hexachlorophene	quinalbarbitone	secobarbital
hexamine hippurate	methenamine hippurate	riboflavine	riboflavin
		sodium calciumedetate	sodium calcium edetate
hydroxyprogesterone hexanoate	hydroxyprogesterone caproate	sodium cromoglycate	sodium cromoglicate
indomethacin	indometacin	sodium ironedetate	sodium feredetate
lysuride	lisuride	sodium picosulphate	sodium picosulfate
methyl cysteine	mecysteine	sorbitan monostearate	sorbitan stearate
methylphenobarbitone	methylphenobarbital	stilboestrol	diethylstilbestrol
oestradiol	estradiol	sulphacetamide	sulfacetamide
oestriol	estriol	sulphadiazine	sulfadiazine
oestrone	estrone	sulphadimidine	sulfadimidine
oxethazaine	oxetacaine	sulphaguanadine	sulfaguanadine
pentaerythritol tetranitrate	pentaerithrityl tetranitrate	sulphamethoxazole	sulfamethoxazole
		sulphasalazine	sulfasalazine
phenobarbitone	phenobarbital	sulphathiazole	sulfathiazole
pipothiazine	pipotiazine	sulphinpyrazone	sulfinpyrazone
polyhexanide	polihexanide	tetracosactrin	tetracosactide
potassium cloazepate	dipotassium clorazepate	thiabendazole	tiabendazole
		thioguanine	tioguanine
pramoxine	pramocaine	thiopentone	thiopental
prothionamide	protionamide	urofollitrophin	urofollitropin

PREFACE

General Practitioners (GPs) are familiar with diagnostic uncertainty, as we deal with illnesses in their earliest presentations. At each consultation we use our knowledge of medicine, of the individual patient, and of his/her social environment to develop the most likely explanation for the consultation. We are aware of the dangers of getting into diagnostic 'ruts' and the need to maintain an open and inquiring mind. Our aspiration is to provide each patient with the best information, in order to facilitate a joint decision about the most appropriate treatment.

Diagnostic uncertainty is not the same as scientific uncertainty. As Naylor observed 'it is easy to confuse personal opinion with evidence or personal ignorance with genuine scientific uncertainty' (*Lancet* 1995; **345**: 840–842). Evidence-based medicine (EBM) is a beacon which helps clarify areas of uncertainty. EBM epitomizes modern general practice and the essence of clinical governance by promoting the most effective care for individual patients.

Evidence-Based Medicine in General Practice is written *by* practising doctors *for* other practising doctors and members of the primary health care team. Both quantitative (numerical) and qualitative (narrative) research is discussed. Each chapter provides a 'working knowledge' of different EBM concepts, illustrated with common examples from general practice. These include the principles of interpreting papers and applying evidence, along with tips on transferring trial findings to individuals and communicating evidence to patients. Although the chapters are designed to 'stand alone' for quick reference, topics are indexed, cross-referenced and include bibliographies to aid further study. The autonomous nature of each chapter means that important principles of EBM are reiterated, giving readers an opportunity to consolidate their EBM skills.

General practice is refreshed by the regular arrival of recently qualified doctors who bring new ideas to complement the experience of existing principles. A new generation of evidence-taught doctors are now joining our profession. This book is designed to help them prepare for the evidence orientated MRCGP exam, and to help those who are already established to develop an appreciation for the benefits that EBM can offer in daily practice.

Many GPs have perceived the evidence-based paradigm as a threat. This book explores the opportunities that EBM offers GPs and their patients. The authors believe that EBM is a powerful tool that can help GPs determine the future of general practice. If our medicine is backed by evidence, then patients, Primary Care Groups and Governments will listen and engage in meaningful debates about health care. The practice of EBM is also fulfilling: it enhances doctor–patient relationships and increases practitioner satisfaction. Read this book and enjoy the results.

Bill Summerskill

Dedicated to Jane and Sean

NATURAL HISTORY OF DISEASE

Roland M. Valori

Most diseases follow a pattern that we call the 'natural history' of disease. When this pattern is entirely predictable it is possible to determine the effects a new treatment has on a disease just by giving the treatment to a sample of patients and comparing the pattern seen to the natural history of the disease. In this situation no control group is necessary because the historical control is sufficiently reliable. There are a few conditions that follow such a predictable course and in some of these it is not necessary to carry out a controlled study, particularly if the condition has a very high mortality, where it might be unethical to have a control group.

The high mortality of untreated meningococcal septicaemia is well known. In the early studies of this condition no control group was required. However, once the first treatment studies showed a reduction in mortality the disease became 'meningococcal septicaemia plus antibiotics', because withholding antibiotics would have been unethical. Thus, a new natural history of disease emerges once a treatment is shown to be effective: the disease modified by the treatment. The control arm of further studies then becomes the disease with the best available treatment.

The controlled trial

In the majority of situations the natural history of disease is variable enough to make it difficult to know whether a treatment is effective or not. This variability is the primary justification for the controlled clinical trial, where the effect of a treatment in one group of patients is compared to the outcome in a group of similar patients who do not receive the treatment. This type of trial tells us whether a treatment improves or worsens the course of an illness. The randomization process adds a refinement to the controlled trial by maximizing the chance that the two experimental groups are the same, by eliminating bias in the selection process. Thus, a randomized controlled trial can be described as an experiment designed to determine the influence of an intervention on the natural history of disease.

Placebo or natural history of disease?

If there is no treatment available for a condition, the control group will not receive active treatment. Because it is recognized that any intervention (even if it is thought to have no biological effect) may modify the natural history of disease, the control group is given a placebo. The purpose of the placebo is to enable the experiment to determine the effect the 'active treatment' has on the disease (its efficacy) independent of the effects of the intervention.

Thus, the placebo arm of the trial becomes the natural history of disease modified by the effect of intervention. This process is not just that of giving a tablet, a sham operation, or a chat in place of a psychological intervention. It also includes the effect of being included in the study (Hawthorne effect). The use of a placebo is to counteract the necessarily artificial nature of the experiment. It can be seen from this that the placebo effect and the natural history of disease become linked, and impossible to separate.

In studies of chronic diseases such as hypertension, migraine and cancer, changes occurring over time in the control group are usually attributed to the placebo effect. However, very often a major component of the change will be the natural history of disease. Authors prefer to refer to the placebo effect even when it is clear the change is due to natural history of disease. The relative contribution of the two effects will depend on the nature of the condition being studied. For example, it is difficult to imagine how a placebo might influence the outcome of cancer, but easier to suppose how it might affect migraine. The important thing to remember is that not all 'placebo effect' is due to the placebo.

Clinical experience *vs.* evidence-based medicine

It is not difficult to see how the natural history of disease and the placebo effect can distort clinical judgement and patient perception of the efficacy of treatment. For example, some people with a sore throat consult their doctor, particularly when their symptoms are at their worst. The natural history of a sore throat is to get better without intervention. If the patient is treated there is a strong likelihood he will get better even if he is a little worse for a while (i.e. even if the peak of his illness is not reached at the time of consultation). Such a positive outcome reinforces the patient's and the doctor's belief that the treatment has had an effect when they are probably experiencing and witnessing natural history of disease. This, in turn, reinforces consultation behaviour, demands for treatment and treatment-giving behaviour (see Example below).

In this example the patient will not usually be harmed. However, use of antibiotics encourages resistant strains to evolve and there is a cost to the health service in doctor-time and treatment. In some situations, failing to appreciate the role of natural history may even lead to the patient being harmed.

Clinical decisions are based on a number of factors, not least the experience of the doctor and his teachers. It can be seen from the example of sore throat that positive change coincident with treatment gives us an **experience** that tells us it is worth using the treatment again in similar situations, even if the treatment is in fact ineffective. If data from a good randomized controlled trial conflict with this experience we can conclude that we did not appreciate the significance of the natural history of disease.

Experience, while extremely important, is nevertheless fallible. However, if there is a conflict of experience and evidence, there remains the possibility that the evidence is not reliable. This is one good reason why it is important to develop skill at searching for and appraising evidence in order to make your own judgement and integrate it with your own experience.

Example

In this randomized controlled trial of antibiotics for sore throat 716 patients with sore throat were randomized to receive immediate antibiotics, delayed antibiotics or no antibiotics (*BMJ* 1997; **315:** 350–352). There was no difference between the antibiotic ($n = 238$) and other groups ($n = 437$) in early returns (5.5 *vs.* 6%) or complications (0.8 *vs.* 0.7%). This indicates that antibiotics did not influence the natural history of sore throat. In contrast, reattendance for future episodes was 38% in the antibiotic group compared to 27% in the other groups. This suggests that giving antibiotics encourages consultation behaviour. Patients were probably encouraged to reattend because of their prior positive experience of improved symptoms with antibiotic use, whereas it is likely that they were just experiencing natural history of disease.

This is an example where explaining the natural history of disease to patients may change expectations and further consultation.

Related topics of interest

DETERMINING CAUSATION

Roland M. Valori

Knowing what causes disease or what causes things to go wrong can help us in a number of ways. It provides us with the means to advise individuals how they might change their behaviour to live more healthily, it allows us to explain adverse reactions to treatment and to direct treatment at the mechanisms underlying disease.

Sometimes there is a single cause for a disorder. More usually there is more than one cause, and often it is only possible to say that a factor contributes to the development of disease. The study designs used to determine causation are similar to those used to assess the benefits and harm of treatment.

Study designs for determining causation

1. Randomized controlled trial.   The randomized controlled trial is the gold standard design for determining causation. Patients are randomized to receive either the putative causative agent or placebo. An example of this type of study is the randomized drug trial. Therapeutic trials will usually compare harmful outcomes between treatment groups, such as the rate of intracerebral bleeding during thrombolysis treatment, as well as positive outcomes. However, such harmful effects of treatment are not usually the primary outcome of the study and the study is rarely large enough to know whether an important difference exists between the groups.

An alternative to the standard therapeutic randomized controlled trial is one that has harm (such as premature death) as the primary outcome. For example a randomized controlled trial could be used to determine the cause of premature death for any number of lifestyle factors such as cholesterol consumption, alcohol, smoking or even riding a bike to work. However, it is usually either unethical or impractical to conduct such studies, so other less precise methods are used.

2. Cohort study.   The second best study design is the cohort study where one of two cohorts are exposed to the putative agent and followed for a period of time. For example, the incidence of new backache at 3 and 12 months postpartum in a group of women who had had epidural analgesia for labour was compared with a group who had not had an epidural (*BMJ* 1996; **312**: 1384–1388). Thus, two cohorts, one with and one without epidural analgesia, were collected at the same point in time (after labour) and assessed prospectively for the development of backache. No difference between the groups was found. The problem with this study design compared to a randomized controlled trial is that the two groups may not be identical and some other factor (perhaps related to the one of interest) not measured in the study may be influencing the outcome.

3. Case–control study.   Both of these study designs pose a question which is answered prospectively and which is therefore less subject to bias. However, these designs are ineffective if the event rate is very low, in which case the best design is the case–controlled study. This type of study uses a retrospective approach that is more prone to bias than its prospective cousins. Nevertheless, for some conditions it is the only choice available and if conducted carefully can provide valuable information on the cause of disease (see related topic: Case–control studies).

Appraisal of studies determining causation

1. Is the study the strongest that could have been performed? Would it be possible and ethical to perform a randomized controlled trial or a cohort study?

2. Were opportunities for exposure and determinants of exposure free from bias? If a study is not randomized it is possible for the groups to be exposed to the risk factor unequally. Alternatively, the measure of exposure may not be objective or it may be subject to recall or other bias. For example retrospective assessment of alcohol or tobacco use can be done objectively, but patients with a disease may recall their lifestyle habits quite differently, particularly if they have already attributed their illness to the factor being studied.

3. Was selection of cases and controls free from bias? This is a particular problem for retrospective studies. Either cases must be sampled randomly or all consecutive cases selected. If a prior association has been identified in a series of patients then patients from this series must not then be included in the study cohort, as this will bias the results. A prior association could have occurred by chance and, if so, this chance association will now inflate the association in the subsequent study. Selection of controls is equally crucial. These must be as similar to the cases as possible to ensure that they have had as much chance of being exposed to the risk factor as the cases.

4. Were both statistical and clinical significance considered? If the odds ratio was not >1, was the sample big enough? In other words, is the event rate sufficiently frequent and is the study sufficiently powered, to determine that a factor is not significantly associated with the outcome of interest?

5. Temporal sequence. Did introduction of the putative agent occur before the outcome of interest?

6. Dose response. Is there a dose–response effect and does the adverse event decrease or disappear when the stimulus is withdrawn?

7. Does the association make sense? Is the association biologically plausible?

8. Consistency. Is this study consistent with other studies?

Example

A prospective cohort study explored the relationship of an employee's control of their job to coronary artery risk (*BMJ* 1997; **314:** 558–565). At baseline a cohort of civil servants was assessed for a number of potential risk factors including low job control. They were reassessed after an average of 5 years for evidence of coronary artery disease. It was found that the odds ratio for subsequent coronary event was 1.93 (CI: 1.34–2.77) for those with low job control. This was unaffected by correction for other known risk factors.

The prospective cohort design is probably the best for this question because it would be unethical to randomize subjects to jobs with low control. The validity of the conclusion depends on two crucial factors. The first is the extent to which the measure 'low job control' is a true measure of low job control and independent of other factors such as low income. The second is how well the outcome measures predict coronary artery disease.

A similar study has shown that high work demand with low economic reward was associated with an objective measure of arterial disease (*Circulation* 1997; **96:** 302–307). It is not difficult to postulate that low job control is associated with high demand/low reward or similar factors. Therefore, it is possible that low job control is a marker for another risk factor. There were four self-reported measures of coronary artery disease. None would be considered a gold standard for evidence of coronary artery disease and self-reporting raises the possibility of reporting bias.

One of the key messages of this study states that 'low job control in the work environment contributes to the development of coronary heart disease among . . .'. The strong implication is that low job control is a causative factor for heart disease. This study has not shown convincingly that job control is a causative factor for coronary artery disease and it could be regarded, at best, as an hypothesis-generating study. Such an hypothesis could be tested in a randomized control trial by randomizing subjects to receive an intervention (aimed at restoring control of their job) or no intervention.

Further reading

Doll R, Peto R. Mortality in relation to smoking: 20 years' observations on male British doctors. *BMJ* 1976; **ii:** 1525–1536.

Sackett DL, Haynes RB, Guyatt GH, Tugwell P. Deciding whether your treatment has done harm. In: *Clinical Epidemiology. A Basic Science for Clinical Medicine.* 2nd edn. Boston/Toronto/London. Little, Brown and Company, 1991, pp. 283–302.

Related topics of interest

OUTCOME MEASURES

Roland M. Valori

In a controlled trial an outcome measure can be any clinical or economic variable relevant to the research question that may be affected by the intervention. Outcome measures are usually divided into primary and secondary. Sometimes secondary outcome measures are further divided into clinical and health economic outcomes.

Primary outcome measure

Normally there will only be one primary outcome measure. This variable will be the single most important outcome of the study, i.e. one that is directly relevant to the research question. It may be a dichotomous outcome, such as alive or dead; a continuous variable such as blood pressure; a questionnaire score, or a health economic outcome such as frequency of consultation or investigation. Sometimes the primary outcome is the time until a particular event such as recurrence of cancer, discharge from hospital or return to work.

It is important for the primary outcome measure to reflect the outcome of the question the study is trying to answer (the research question). For example, frequency of stroke would be the primary outcome measure in a study of carotid endarterectomy for prevention of stroke. A further consideration is the care with which the outcome is defined. In this example minor transient strokes might be common but not clinically important and therefore outside the definition of the primary outcome. The ability to define the primary outcome measure will depend on the wording of the research question. However, a clearly worded question does not guarantee a perfectly defined outcome measure. Care must be exercised with both.

1. Timing. The timing of the outcome measure is important. Some interventions may exert a short-term benefit that is gradually eroded over time (see example). Alternatively some treatments are given for prolonged periods and their beneficial effect may not be apparent in the early phase of treatment. For practical reasons it is difficult to maintain data monitoring beyond one or two years. Therefore, the literature is biased towards studies that are able to measure outcomes over a relatively short period of time.

2. Surrogate outcomes. Occasionally events of clinical importance are so rare that surrogate markers of outcome are used. In studies of cytoprotection of NSAIDs, endoscopically proven ulcers (which are quite common) are used as surrogates for peptic ulcer bleeding or perforation (which are very rare). Care must be taken with surrogate markers because they cannot always be relied upon to predict the outcome for which they have been substituted. One of the best examples of this problem is a study of the use of lipid-lowering agent clofibrate for primary prevention of ischaemic heart disease (*Lancet* 1984; **ii:** 600–604). Cholesterol level was the primary outcome measure. It was used as a surrogate for cardiovascular morbidity and mortality. A significant reduction in cholesterol and non-fatal myocardial infarction were demonstrated but there were 47% more deaths in the clofibrate group during the treatment period. Thus, the increase in all-cause mortality overwhelmed any positive effects clofibrate had on cholesterol or non-fatal cardiac events (*Lancet* 1984; **ii:** 600–604). More recent studies of lipid-lowering agents use cardiovascular-related morbidity or mortality as the primary outcome measure.

3. Sample size calculation. A very important aspect of the primary outcome is the calculation of sample size. Sample size calculations are done to determine how many subjects are required in a study to be certain of the outcome. Certainty in this context refers to a reasonable certainty that an important difference has not been missed because too few patients were included in the study. There are two characteristics of the primary outcome measure that affect sample size: variability and the size of change that is thought to be clinically important. The more variable the outcome measure, the greater the sample size. If only a small difference in the primary outcome is considered important then a larger sample size is needed to be certain that a difference is not missed.

Secondary outcome measures

Secondary outcome measures include all other variables that are considered important to the research question. This might include drug side effects, complications of surgical interventions, quality-of-life measures, satisfaction rating scales and a great variety of health economic outcomes. Secondary outcome measures paint a much broader picture of the effects of the intervention and no study would be complete without them. However, too much emphasis can be placed on secondary outcome measures, particularly if no change is observed in the primary outcome.

The commonest error is to start searching (fishing) for statistically significant differences between groups. A significant difference at the 5% level (*P*<0.05) will be found by chance with 1 in 20 variables. Therefore, if multiple comparisons are made, a statistical correction (such as a Bonferroni correction) for multiple tests should be used. Another error is to infer there are no differences between groups when there might be. The sample size is based on the primary outcome measure and it is likely that the sample size for the secondary outcomes (particularly rare ones such as complications or side effects) will be too small to decide with certainty that there is no difference between groups (type II error).

Appraisal tips

1. Be suspicious if there is no primary outcome measure or if there is more than one.
2. Try to determine whether the primary outcome measure truly reflects the research question and whether it is sufficiently focused to be clinically useful.
3. Beware of surrogate measures.
4. If the measure is not objective or clear cut, try to determine whether the assessor(s) were truly blind to the allocation.
5. For secondary measures try to decide whether all the important variables were considered.
6. Do not forget how difficult trials are to do, and that there is a balance between what is desirable and what is feasible to measure.

7. Finally, beware of excessive analysis of secondary outcome measures: they are there to paint a broad picture, not to answer a specific research question.

Example

The Diabetes Control and Complications Trial (DCCT; *New England Journal of Medicine* 1993; **329:** 977–986) was designed to determine the effects of tight glycaemic control on microvascular end points in insulin-dependent diabetes. The principal endpoint was development and progression of retinopathy with secondary endpoints of other microvascular disease (neuropathy and nephropathy) and macrovascular disease (cardiovascular disease).

The DCCT showed significant reductions in all of the microvascular endpoints and was a landmark trial in this respect. These are very clinically significant outcomes for individuals with diabetes. They represent a reduction in development of blindness, need for dialysis and the numbness and pain often endured by long-term diabetics. However, the reduction in cardiovascular (macrovascular) disease was not significant (41% drop in CVD events (95 CI – 10 ± 68%)). The failure to show a significant change in cardiovascular disease should not be interpreted as a lack of effect as the study was not powered on this endpoint and in fact had relatively young participants at low CVS risk. Furthermore, the lack of evidence for this endpoint should be balanced against the overwhelming evidence for the other outcomes.

Further reading

Bowling A. *Measuring disease.* Milton Keynes, Oxford University Press, 1996.

Guyatt GH, Feeny DH, Patrick DL. Measuring health-related quality of life. *Annals of Internal Medicine*, 1993; **118:** 622–629.

Wilkin D, Hallam L, Doggett MA. *Measures of need and outcome for primary care.* Oxford, England, Oxford University Press, 1992.

Related topics of interest

Formulating clinical questions (p. 10); Randomized controlled trials (p. 25); Critical appraisal (p. 70); Bias and confounders (p. 101); The power of studies (p. 108); Subgroup analysis (p. 117); Improving professional practice (p. 142).

FORMULATING CLINICAL QUESTIONS

Marcel Levi

One of the hardest steps in practising evidence-based medicine may be the translation of a clinical (patient) problem into an answerable clinical question. Regardless of whether the patient problem is about the optimal diagnostic approach, the optimal therapeutic strategy or even prognosis, the definition and structure of an appropriate clinical question is crucial in order to successfully find the appropriate evidence for solving that problem.

Why should we ask an answerable clinical question?

There are several reasons why we should construct answerable clinical questions:

1. Formulating a clinical question focuses attention to the real (clinical) problem at hand and will ultimately lead to the evidence relevant to the problem.
2. The appropriate definition of a clinical question provides guidance as to where to find evidence that is relevant to the question.
3. The properly formulated clinical question will suggest the format of the answer, and also suggest the type of evidence that should be sought.

How to formulate an answerable clinical question?

The answerable clinical question should contain three or four key elements:

1. The **patient** (category) in question.
2. The diagnostic or therapeutic **intervention**.
3. The intervention that is taken as a **comparison** to the intervention in statement 2 (could be placebo).
4. The **outcome**.

Example

You receive a letter from outpatients regarding a 68-year-old female patient with type II diabetes who has been found to have a loud systolic murmur over the right carotid artery on routine physical examination. The hospital team have organized a carotid Doppler showing a > 90% stenosis of the carotid artery and request that you refer her to a vascular surgeon. The patient attends your surgery the following week and you discuss the situation with her. She has no neurologic complaints or symptoms and asks whether she really needs an operation (a carotid endarterectomy). She is frightened by the prospect of surgery but has heard that she may have a stroke if she waits. You decide to find out the risk of developing an ischaemic stroke in this patient with or without the operation.

The '**patient**' in this clinical question could be 'a patient with a severe, but asymptomatic, carotid artery stenosis'. The '**intervention**' is 'carotid artery endarterectomy'. In this example no '**comparison intervention**' has been mentioned, but it could have been something like 'medical treatment' (such as aspirin or a cholesterol lowering agent). The '**outcome**' may be defined as 'the risk of ischaemic stroke', taking into account the peri-operative risk and the long-term outcome.

Taken together, this problem could result in an answerable clinical question such as: **What is the effect of a carotid endarterectomy on the peri-operative and long-term incidence of ischaemic stroke in an asymptomatic patient with a severe stenosis of the carotid artery.**

Preciseness of the question

From the above example it is clear that when defining the key elements in the clinical question several choices can be made. The degree of detail in the chosen definitions will play an important role in the kind of answer that will be retrieved. If one limits the patient category to 'a 62-year-old female diabetic patient with an asymptomatic carotid artery stenosis' the yielded evidence would be highly applicable to that patient. However, the chances are high that there will not be very specific information as a result of choosing this narrowly defined patient category. Conversely, if 'all patients with a carotid artery stenosis' become the question subject, there will probably be a considerable amount of literature, but it is likely that much of this literature will not strictly be applicable to this patient. For example, it may be that all retrieved evidence comes from clinical studies in which only men (and only a few diabetics) were included. How relevant the results from these studies would be in this situation is a difficult question to answer. This is dealt with elsewhere in the book (see Related topics).

Definition of the outcome requires similar choices. Although in the example 'ischaemic stroke' was chosen as the most appropriate end-point, it might well be that from a patient's perspective 'long-term neurologic deficit' or 'all cardiovascular morbidity and mortality' might be more relevant.

Potential pitfalls in constructing questions

There are a number of potential pitfalls that need to be considered when translating clinical problems into well-formulated clinical questions:

1. The problem may be too complicated or there may be too many questions to be answered in a given clinical situation. One solution may be to focus on the question that is most relevant to the patient and/or is most likely to generate an appropriate answer.
2. To be able to formulate a relevant question and to make the appropriate choices for the various components of the question, sufficient background knowledge may be required. For example, to choose how specific the 'patient' in the example above needs to be defined, it is important to have a general idea whether men have different outcomes from women in carotid stenosis (this, of course, generates further clinical questions) or whether 'diabetes' will seriously affect the outcome.
3. There are always more questions than time available to find answers to them. It has been estimated that during an average working week, a practising physician will encounter approximately 60 clinical questions that need to be answered. Again, the solution may be important to focus on the questions that are most relevant to the most important clinical situations.

Further reading

Richardson WS, *et al.* The well-built clinical question: a key to evidence-based decisions. *ACP J Club* 1995; **123:** A12–13.

Smith R. What clinical information do doctors need? *BMJ* 1996; **313:** 1062–1068.

Related topics of interest

Search strategies for electronic databases (p. 63); Sampling and applicability (p. 130).

HIERARCHY OF EVIDENCE

William S.M. Summerskill

Willie Sutton robbed over 100 banks in America. When asked 'why?' he is credited with the reply: 'because that's where the money is'. Like financial wealth, statistical wealth is concentrated in centres of power. In most clinical situations, the value of evidence is directly proportional to the statistical power of the study. This allows the construction of a hierarchy of evidence based on the strength of different study designs to answer specific research questions.

Definition

The hierarchy of evidence is a spectrum of potential sources, beginning with those most likely to provide the best evidence. The extent of the list will depend upon the clinical question addressed. Randomized controlled trials are best for assessing interventions; cohort and case–control studies are useful for answering questions about causation. For qualitative questions, a phenomenological study of six patients experiencing a specific situation may be at the apex of the evidence list. The object of an evidence hierarchy is to follow Sutton's example and concentrate one's efforts on the sources most likely to yield rewards.

Quantitative research

For the majority of quantitative questions, the hierarchy parallels statistical power, as illustrated in Figure 1. In this idealized 'pecking order' of published, peer-reviewed studies, the apex is occupied by systematic reviews including meta-analyses. The greatest statistical certainty comes from well-conducted meta-analyses that incorporate a number of RCTs. Because of the large number of participants involved in meta-analyses, the results are more generalizable to populations. Conversely, trial designs further down the pyramid produce results that are less readily translated to other populations, but may be more applicable to specific types of patients. A special consideration is the $n = 1$ trial, which some investigators place at the apex because they yield highly personalized evidence.

Similar hierarchies are applied to discriminate recommendations for clinical practice. Figure 2 is adapted from the North of England evidence-based guideline project (*BMJ* 1998; **316:** 1332–1335) – a grade IV recommendation! The greater the predictive power of the trial design, the higher the resulting recommendations are valued. Recommendations are given alphabetical grades A–D, corresponding to evidence categories I–IV. Hence, interventions based on a cohort study would be referred to as grade 'B' recommendations as they reflect category II evidence. Consensus statements are common forms of clinical recommendation, but their unsystematic design is most influenced by bias and least directed by evidence.

Using the evidence hierarchy

Although size and fitness are good indicators of performance in sporting events, the strongest team does not always win. Hierarchies are guides to relative statistical size and methodological fitness, but they do not account for the quality of individual

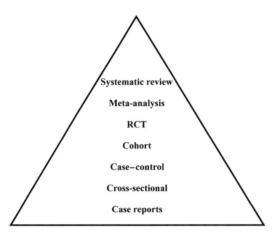

Figure 1. Hierarchy of evidence in quantitative studies.

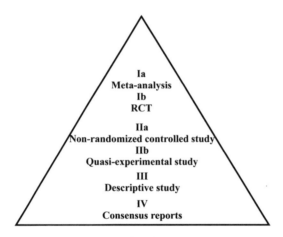

Figure 2. Categories of evidence.

trials. There can be overlap at any level, so that a well-designed RCT can be more useful than a mediocre meta-analysis. Therefore identifying a meta-analysis or RCT is not a surrogate for confirming the validity of its findings.

The hierarchy does not exclude data from other sources. Instead it provides an idealized target for the efficient retrieval of relevant studies. In some situations, there may be no meta-analyses or RCTs. The hierarchy then serves to guide clinicians in an ordered manner to the best available evidence, based on the reliability of that particular study design. Conversely, when many sources of potential evidence are available, the hierarchy provides a guide to those sources likely to be most informative.

In either situation, trial design can be used as a search tool to find articles when information seems scanty, or to filter studies when excessive numbers of articles are found. Such strategies should be explicitly stated and explained in any review. Evidence from a case report becomes more significant when it can be demonstrated that thorough searches failed to identify any trials higher than this in the evidence hierarchy. However, a case report is a weak source of evidence if appropriate meta-analyses and RCTs on the same subject have not been considered.

Qualitative research

The evidence hierarchy in qualitative research is not fixed, but is constructed on the basis of methodological reliability to yield answers to the clinical question. The order is more fluid, as the best source of evidence for any particular question will be determined by the information required. Like quantitative research, the ideal study may not have been performed, so the same process of tier-by-tier searching is required until the best available evidence is found.

Further reading

Guyatt GH, Haynes RB, Jaeschke RZ, Cook DJ, Green L, Naylor CD, Wilson MC, Richardson WS. Users' guides to the medical literature: XXV. Evidence-based medicine: Principles for applying the users' guides to patient care. *JAMA* 2000; **284:** 1290–1296.
Shekelle PG, Woolf SH, Eccles M, Grimshaw J. Developing Guidelines. *BMJ* 1999; **318:** 593–596.

Related topics of interest

Systematic reviews (p. 16); Meta-analyses (p. 19); Randomized controlled trials (p. 25); Cohort studies (p. 33); Case–control studies (p. 37); Cross-sectional (prevalence) surveys (p. 41); Case reports and case series (p. 44); Qualitative research (p. 46); Search strategies for electronic databases (p. 63); The power of studies (p. 108).

SYSTEMATIC REVIEWS

Dermot P.B. McGovern

Reviews are potentially a good source of information for busy healthcare professionals, as, in theory at least; they should provide a summary of all the studies addressing a single clinical question. However many reviews are written by 'experts' within the particular field who present their own collection of papers or promote their own research. These sorts of reviews are often biased and may be misleading. The rationale for systematic reviews is to provide unbiased summaries of all the available evidence thus avoiding these potential pitfalls. To achieve this systematic reviews are executed according to very strictly defined and reproducible methodologies.

Basic structure of a systematic review

Systematic reviews should set out to address a clearly defined and appropriate clinical question. This should be followed by an exhaustive search of the literature to identify relevant studies that address this question. Strict and reproducible criteria for study inclusion in the review should be stipulated and the results (summary) of the review should be presented in an unbiased fashion.

Important methodological issues

The principles and basic structure of systematic reviews are simple enough, but there are plenty of potential pitfalls for researchers undertaking these analyses:

1. The researchers may not be asking a clinically relevant problem. The results of the review may then be interesting as an academic exercise, but of no real relevance to everyday practice.
2. One of the fundamental principles of systematic reviews is that they should be based upon an exhaustive search of the literature. This should, as standard, include:
   - Searches of all the electronic databases;
   - Searches of the www;
   - Searches through other reviews addressing the same subject;
   - 'Experts' within the field can be contacted (identified via the National Research Register, UK) and asked if they know of any other relevant studies;
   - Search for unpublished data;
   - Searches of the 'grey' literature (internal reports, pharmaceutical industry data, non-peer-reviewed journals). The SIGLE database is useful for this;
   - Searches of the bibliography of all identified articles;
   - Authors of published data should be contacted for missing information;
   - Cochrane controlled clinical trials register.

   One of the major problems of reviews is that of '**publication bias**'. Studies are far more likely to be published if they contain positive results (authors are probably more enthusiastic about getting them into print and editors feel that studies with positive results are more likely to be cited). A recent review examining systematic reviews and the 'grey literature' (unpublished studies) suggested that in only a third of meta-analyses was the grey literature searched and that published work showed a larger estimate of intervention effect (odds ratio 1.15 (1.04–1.28)) than unpublished data.

Searches should not be restricted to English language papers/journals only. There is evidence that studies with positive results from Germany are more likely to be published in English than negative studies, which are more likely to be published in German.

3. Reviews are only as good as the studies they have included. The primary studies should all address the clinical question that the review is attempting to resolve. These individual studies should have undergone a rigorous quality control exercise before inclusion in the review. Inclusion criteria should be clearly defined and agreed upon prospectively. It is reassuring to see more than one person decide upon inclusion, ideally blind to other people's assessment. It is even more reassuring to see a high degree of agreement on inclusion/exclusion of studies thus proving the robustness of the entry criteria. The methods for resolving inclusion/exclusion disputes should be clearly stated. A process where good studies carry more 'weight' towards the overall results than an indifferent study is one way of coping with variable study quality.

4. Presentation of results in a review can often be difficult. If the review includes quantitative studies (especially randomized controlled trials) then it is standard to perform a meta-analysis (a statistical analysis which 'pools' the data from the primary studies). Qualitative data can be more difficult to summarize and sometimes there is no meaningful way to combine the study results. It may be that the summary becomes the authors' subjective view of the evidence. It is important for people reading reviews to assess whether they believe that the author's summary is representative of the evidence put forward in the review.

5. Is there evidence of heterogeneity in the results? This is covered in detail in the chapter on meta-analysis.

6. Are the results applicable to your patient? This will depend on the individual study inclusion/exclusion criteria. A good question to ask is 'would my patient 'pass' the inclusion/exclusion criteria of most of the studies?'. If the answer is yes then the results can probably be applied to your patient. If not then ask yourself if your patient is so different from those included in the study, thus making the study conclusions irrelevant or are the differences minor and can they be ignored? The answer to the generalizability/applicability of review results usually comes down to clinical judgement.

Advantages of systematic reviews (these equally apply to meta-analyses)

1. 'Tight' methodology eliminates bias.
2. Convenient amalgamation of large amounts of data which can be rapidly 'digested' by healthcare workers.
3. Pooling of data empowers the research and therefore
   - Beneficial effects of interventions may be 'discovered' sooner.
   - The results are more precise (as shown by narrower confidence intervals than those in the primary studies).
4. Heterogeneity between primary studies identifies new avenues of research.

Quality control questions for systematic reviews

1. Is a clinically relevant and well-defined question being asked?
2. Were the search methods described exhaustive?
3. How was the quality of the primary studies assessed? Was there a weighting system/rejection of poor quality studies?
4. Was missing information sought?
5. Was heterogeneity of effect investigated? (See chapter on meta-analysis.)
6. Do the conclusions reflect the evidence?
7. Are the results generalizable to your patient?

Example (Systematic review of near patient test evaluations in primary care. *BMJ* 1999; 319: 824–827)

This systematic review had a clear objective of identifying and qualitatively synthesizing the findings of all studies that have examined the performance and effect of near patient tests in the primary care setting. They performed an extensive search using five electronic databases, a hand search of trade journals and primary care conference proceedings and also contacted researchers and commercial organizers with an interest in the field. The authors also examined the references of all identified articles.

The authors identified 101 appropriate publications. They evaluated the quality of these through the use of prospectively stipulated criteria and found the studies to be generally of poor quality. As a result only 32 papers were reviewed in detail. There was some evidence of benefit of near patient testing in anticoagulant monitoring and testing for group A β-haemolytic streptococcus. However the authors found disagreement or inconsistent reference standards in the effectiveness of near patient urine dipstick testing for urinary tract infection and near patient tests for *Helicobacter pylori* respectively. The authors also felt that they found no evidence of unbiased assessment of the effect of near patient tests in primary care on patient outcomes, organizational outcomes or cost. The results of this study demonstrate the difficulty sometimes experienced in coming to a sensible conclusion of a systematic review. Furthermore given the quality of the data it would have been very difficult and inappropriate to attempt a formal pooled statistical analysis. Despite an appropriate search the authors had to conclude that:

- There is little evidence to promote the expansion of near patient testing in primary care.
- Further research was needed.

Further reading

Greenlagh T. Papers that summarise other papers (systematic reviews and meta-analyses). *BMJ* 1997; **315:** 672–675.

Related topics of interest

Meta-analyses (p. 19); Sources of information (p. 57); Relative risk, relative risk reduction and odds ratio (p. 79); Risk reduction and the number needed to treat (NNT) (p. 83).

META-ANALYSES

Dermot P.B. McGovern

Many of the principles that apply to meta-analyses are applicable to systematic reviews and it will be useful to read the chapter about systematic reviews prior to reading this chapter.

A meta-analysis is the mathematical sum of the results of more than one primary study, all of which have used similar methods in order to address the same question. Meta-analyses are often presented as the statistical analysis (where appropriate) of a systematic review but may also be studies in their own right. The basic principles that apply to systematic reviews are also relevant to meta-analyses, namely that the studies should include:

- A thorough search of the literature.
- Explicit and sound study inclusion/exclusion criteria.

For more information on the methods for a comprehensive search of the literature and assessing trials for inclusion/exclusion from the review please refer to the chapter on systematic reviews.

The results of the studies included in a meta-analysis are usually presented in a standard form – the forest plot. A theoretical example of a forest plot is given in Figure 1.

The horizontal lines on a forest plot represent the (95%) confidence intervals of the results (odds ratio or relative risk) from each study. The shaded shape at the centre of each line represents the point estimate of the odds ratio from that trial (i.e. the actual 'result' of the trial). The central vertical line represents the line of no effect usually equal to an odds ratio/relative risk of 1.0. If a study point estimate rests on the line then there is no difference in efficacy between the two treatments. If a point estimate lies to the left of the line of no effect this study favours treatment A (studies a, c, d, e and g) and if it lies to the right it favours treatment B (studies b

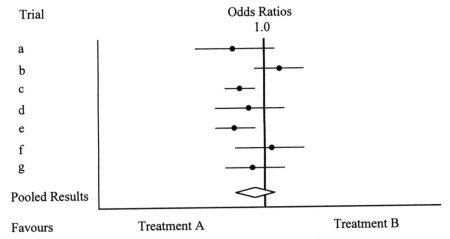

Figure 1. A theoretical forest plot showing the results of a meta-analysis comparing Treatment A and B. The individual trials are listed on the left hand side and their results are represented by the dark circles and horizontal lines. The diamond represents the pooled results of all included studies.

and f). However if the horizontal line representing the (95%) confidence intervals crosses the line of no effect (studies a, b, d, f and g) then there is no statistically significant difference between the two treatments ($P > 0.05$). The diamond at the bottom of the graph represents the pooled data for all studies and the width of the diamond represents the confidence limits that are much narrower than those of the individual studies as a result of the increased number of study participants and hence increased power of this analysis. The same principles regarding position in relation to the line of no effect apply to the results of the pooled data.

Heterogeneity

This is an important concept to understand when reading a meta-analysis. A glance at the forest plot of any study will show if all the horizontal lines (representing the confidence limits) overlap to some degree. If they do then homogeneity of the results is said to be present and the results of each trial are compatible with the results from all the others. This is the case in the theoretical example in Figure 1. If any of the lines do not overlap with any of the others then heterogeneity is said to be present (see Figure 2). That is, from study to study, there is greater variation in the results than can be expected by chance alone. This implies that the trials are significantly different in some respect (population, data collection, trial design etc.) and that the results should probably not be pooled and presented as one overall figure. If heterogeneity is present then this should open a new line of enquiry as to why the treatment is more/less effective in certain subgroups. This identification of potentially significant clinical subsets is one of the strengths of meta-analysis. There are statistical tests (variations of the chi-squared test) that can test for heterogeneity but on the whole these tests are not robust.

The results of meta-analyses are usually expressed as odds ratios or relative risks. The odds ratio will closely equate to the relative risk as long as the outcome occurs infrequently ($< 20\%$). If the outcome occurs more frequently than this then the odds ratio will overestimate the relative risk. If the meta-analysis is asking a question about interventions it is more useful to calculate the

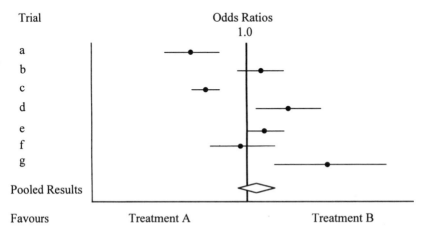

Figure 2. Theoretical meta-analysis comparing treatment A and B. This forest plot suggests heterogeneity across the trials. Note that the 95% confidence intervals for study a do not overlap with those of study b, d, e or g.

20 META-ANALYSES

numbers needed to treat (NNT) or harm (NNH) and this can be done simply and is demonstrated in the chapter on NNT/NNH.

Sensitivity analysis

There is more than one correct method of performing a meta-analysis and it is important to assess how sensitive or robust the results of any meta-analysis are to any change in study methodology. This process is called a sensitivity analysis and re-analysis of the data can occur in a variety of settings including:

- Use of alternative statistical models.
- Alternative study inclusion criteria (e.g. only including very high quality studies or inclusion of more substandard studies).
- Exclusion of unpublished studies.
- Inclusion of patients lost to follow-up and assigning them to the 'worst case scenario'.

If the results remain consistent despite these manipulations then one can be more confident about their reliability. A good example of where a sensitivity analysis has made a difference to the results of a meta-analysis is in a review of the effectiveness of mammography for breast cancer screening published in the *Lancet* (see Further reading). The review argues that six of the randomized trials have flaws in their randomization process. When an analysis is only performed on the 'good' trials no benefit from breast cancer screening is seen (relative risk for death from breast cancer 1.04 (95% CI 0.85 to 1.25)) in contrast to the benefit seen when the six 'bad' trials are included giving a relative risk of 0.80 (95% CI 0.73 to 0.88). This study is discussed further in the chapter on screening.

Meta-analyses are not universally regarded as the studies at the peak of the hierarchy of evidence. For example an infamous meta-analysis demonstrated that intravenous magnesium was effective in acute myocardial infarction. A subsequent very large, multi-centre, randomized controlled trial (ISIS 4) however, showed no benefit (arguments still persist about the timing of the infusion!) and re-analysis of the original meta-analysis demonstrated some fundamental methodological flaws.

Opponents of meta-analyses often quote this example as proof of the fallibility of meta-analysis, however it is important to remember that if any study (RCT, meta-analysis, observational study etc.) is poorly conducted then the results are likely to be flawed. Other commentators have stated that it is intrinsically wrong to pool the results of trials that were probably performed on different populations, under different circumstances with different methods. Others simply feel that if a meta-analysis is needed to demonstrate the effectiveness of an intervention then it is probably not effective enough to warrant a change to clinical practice.

As increasing numbers of meta-analyses are performed, it will become increasingly likely to find more than one meta-analysis/systematic review addressing a clinical question. This is fine if the studies' conclusions agree. What if they don't? The first check should be to use the meta-analysis 'quality control' questions (see below) to identify potential problems of study methodology. Meta-analyses on the same subject may come to differing answers if they have slightly different study inclusion and exclusion criteria. A recent example of this occurred when the *BMJ* published a meta-analysis of anticoagulation in non-rheumatic atrial fibrillation, which found no benefit. However fairly recently a meta-analysis on the same subject came to the opposite conclusion. The main difference between the studies was the exclusion of one large study from the second analysis (see Further reading). In theory meta-analyses answering the same question and using the standard methods should come to the same statistical conclusion. Systematic reviews without a meta-analysis (e.g. asking a question which requires qualitative data) rely more on the author's subjective view to provide a conclusion. Do the conclusions reflect the data presented? If the conclusions of reviews differ and there is no obvious reason for this then most people would agree it would be valid to identify the RCT whose inclusion/exclusion criteria most 'fit' your patient in order to answer your question.

Assessing a meta-analysis

When reading a meta-analysis the following questions should be asked in order to assess the validity of the study results:

1. Is the clinical question well defined?
2. Was there a thorough search and did the authors chase missing data?
3. Were the individual study designs reviewed and were the trials weighted accordingly?
4. Was heterogeneity analyzed?
5. Was an appropriate sensitivity analysis performed?
6. Are the stated conclusions reasonable and do they reflect the study results?

Example (Risk of gastrointestinal haemorrhage with long term use of aspirin: meta-analysis. *BMJ* 2000; 321: 1183–1187)

This meta-analysis assessed the risk of gastrointestinal haemorrhage with long-term use of aspirin. The authors posed a clear clinical question: their aim was to 'assess the incidence of gastrointestinal haemorrhage associated with long term aspirin therapy and to determine the effect of dose reduction and formulation on the incidence of such haemorrhage'.

The authors took advantage of a previously conducted meta-analysis and performed an adequate search (both electronic and manual), using appropriate free text terms. Reassuringly their search overlapped by three years with the previous meta-analysis and they neither missed nor 'found' any relevant studies. They did not limit their search to English language publications. There is however no mention of chasing any missing data. They included 24 randomized controlled trials (containing approximately 66 000 patients) although some of these were not placebo-controlled.

- The authors independently reviewed the design and quality of all studies but no statistical analysis on their disagreement/agreement concordance was performed. No weighting according to study quality was performed.
- The authors state that no significant heterogeneity was observed but do not expand on this statement. 'Eyeballing' the forest plot (Figure 3) confirms that there is no apparent heterogeneity.
- A sensitivity analysis was performed where the authors excluded the two largest studies to

check that these did not have undue influence on the overall results. No sensitivity analysis was performed removing studies of inferior design etc.

- The results show that the pooled odds ratio for gastrointestinal haemorrhage with aspirin was 1.68 (95% confidence interval 1.51 to 1.88). The numbers needed to harm (NNH) (based on an average 28 months of aspirin) was 106 (95% CI 82 to 140). The authors also looked specifically at the subgroups of low dose aspirin (50–162.5 mg/day) and modified release formulations. The results remained statistically significant with pooled odds ratios of 1.59 (1.40 to 1.81) and 1.93 (1.15 to 3.23) respectively.
- The discussion gives a well-balanced account of the risks and benefits of aspirin therapy and certainly reflects the data presented.

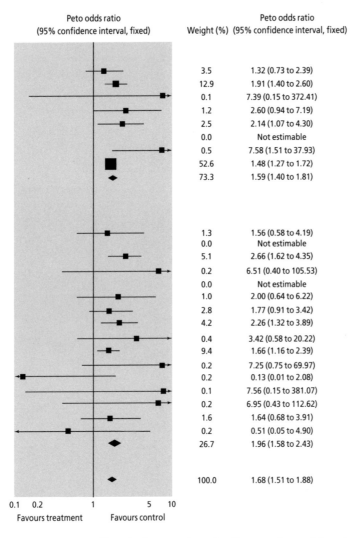

Figure 3. Peto odds ratio for gastrointestinal haemorrhage with aspirin (Reprinted from *BMJ* volume 321, 11 November 2000 with permission of the BMJ Publishing group).

Further reading

Gotzsche PC, Olsen O. Is screening for breast cancer with mammography justifiable? *Lancet* 2000; **355:** 129–134.

Greenlagh T. Papers that summarise other papers (systematic reviews and meta-analyses). *BMJ* 1997; **315:** 672–675.

Related topics of interest

Hierarchy of evidence (p. 13); Systematic reviews (p. 16); Relative risk, relative risk reduction and odds ratio (p. 79); Risk reduction and the number needed to treat (NNT) (p. 83).

RANDOMIZED CONTROLLED TRIALS

Dermot P.B. McGovern

The randomized controlled trial (RCT) has, in some ways, become the talisman for the EBM movement and is regarded, by many, as the gold standard trial for evaluating therapeutic interventions. The RCT came into being as it became obvious (to Pierre Louis and others in 19th century Paris) that observation of, and anecdotal reporting of, the results of therapeutic trials was inherently flawed. The fundamental problems of these 'trials' were the lack of a control group and the almost inevitability of bias.

Basic 'structure' of RCTs

The overall structure of an RCT is summarized in Figure 1. In Figure 1 and the rest of this chapter only trials of two groups are discussed. RCTs can theoretically contain an infinite number of groups as long as the basic 'rules' are adhered to.

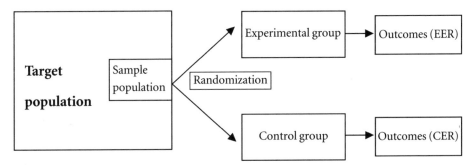

Figure 1. Diagrammatic representation of a (randomized) controlled trial. EER – Experimental Event Rate CER – Control Event Rate.

A sample of a target population is randomized to receive the trial therapy (**intervention** or **experimental group**) or not (**control group**). The two groups are treated and observed in an identical fashion. The groups are followed for a specified length of time at which point the trial ends. Data can be analyzed as the trial proceeds or at the end of the trial. The results from the intervention group are compared with those from the control group and as the groups should otherwise have been treated identically, any differences in outcomes are attributed to the trial therapy.

Finer points of RCT methods

A sample of patients is taken from the target population; the important 'outcome' of this step is that the sample should be representative of the target population as a whole. Potential recruits for the trials are identified and their eligibility is judged against the study inclusion/exclusion criteria. These criteria determine the ultimate generalizability and validity of the trial. Patients are included in the trials following informed consent. The majority of medical journals will not include studies that do not have ethics committee approval, which includes an evaluation of the quality of informed consent.

Randomization of trial participants is included to ensure that the two groups are similar for important baseline characteristics enabling outcomes to be attributed to the trial therapy and not to intrinsically dissimilar groups. Tables comparing the baseline characteristics of the two groups are often presented early in RCT reports. Some authorities believe that randomization leading to similar groups depends to a degree on luck and patients should in fact be stratified (placed into sub-groups) for important characteristics thus 'ensuring' similar groups. Randomization may, however, also match groups for unknown confounders. Randomization can either occur individually (e.g. by post-code, date of birth, random number generator) or at group level (e.g. randomization of communities).

The **control group's** role is to act as a 'baseline' or comparison group for the intervention group. The two groups should be treated identically (including methods of data extraction) except that the intervention group should receive trial therapy and the control group should 'receive' one of the following:

- **Nothing** – Participants may not even know that they are part of a trial.
- **Observation** – People behave differently when they are included in a trial (Hawthorne effect). Observing the control group in an identical fashion ensures that outcome differences are not due to behavioural differences.
- **Placebo** – Placebos are 'dummy', inert pills or solutions that appear identical to the trial therapy. Inclusion of placebos helps 'control' for the 'placebo effect'.
- **Gold standard therapy** – It may be unethical to treat patients with placebo (e.g. acute myocardial infarction). Furthermore significant advances are achieved when novel therapies are found to be superior to existing ones.

Studies can be **single-blinded** (patient alone unaware of whether in active or control group), **double-blinded** (both patient and doctor unaware) or **open-label** (everyone aware). 'Blinding' avoids the effect of bias but is not always possible (i.e. comparison of laparoscopic with open cholecystectomy). Analysis of the results should relate to appropriate **outcomes** with relevance to everyday clinical practice. All patients who entered the study should be included in the analysis and analyzed in the group they were originally allocated to no matter what has actually gone on in the trial (i.e. died, poor compliance, received wrong treatment etc.). This type of analysis reflects everyday clinical practice and is called an **intention to treat analysis** (as opposed to a completed treatment analysis).

The data may be analyzed in patient sub-groups. These analyses should be treated with caution:

- Analysis of retrospectively assigned sub-groups should be regarded as 'fishing' for positive results. One authority has suggested that retrospective subgroup analysis can best be summed up with the following analogy: If a man goes fishing and catches a boot he should throw it back and not pretend that he was fishing for boots all along.
- Sub-groups **prospectively** assigned for good biological reasons are less frowned upon but the results should be corrected for multiple testing (i.e. the more

questions you ask the more likely you are to get a positive result if conventional levels of statistical significance are used).

An infamous retrospective sub-group analysis 'demonstrated' that patients born under the astrological birth signs of Libra or Gemini are unlikely to benefit from aspirin in acute myocardial infarction.

Disadvantages of controlled trials

The most limiting disadvantage of properly conducted (randomized) controlled trials is that they are expensive as large numbers of patients and prolonged follow up and recruitment time are usually needed. Funding for these trials is often difficult to obtain except with the support of a pharmaceutical company (which may bring its own particular problems).

Evaluating a controlled trial

When evaluating a controlled trial the following questions will help assess its methodology and thus whether its results can be trusted.

1. Were patients randomized to treatments and were investigators and patients blind to the randomization process?
2. Were the groups similar for important prognostic characteristics at the start of the trial?
3. Were the patients analyzed in the groups to which they were allocated?
4. Were all the patients accounted for at the end of the trial?
5. Were the groups treated equally, apart from receiving the trial therapy (or not) throughout the trial?
6. Were all clinically appropriate outcomes measured?
7. Can the results of this study be extrapolated to my patients?
8. Did an ethics committee approve the trial and who funded it?

If the trial methodology is sound it is important to consider whether any statistically significant results are clinically significant. It is also important to note if the treatment caused any significant adverse events.

Example (Randomised trial of cholesterol lowering in 4444 patients with coronary heart disease: the Scandinavian Simvastatin Survival Study (4S). *Lancet* 1994: 344; 1383–1389)

A total of 4444 patients were recruited as the **sample population** meant to represent the **target population** of patients with coronary heart disease (CHD) and serum cholesterol in the range of 5.5–8.0 mmol/l. A number of appropriate **exclusion criteria** including planned coronary artery surgery, congestive heart failure and child-bearing potential were applied. The study **intervention** was the HMG-CoA reductase inhibitor simvastatin and the **comparator** was an appropriate placebo. The patients were **randomized** to treatment or placebo group but only after **stratification** for previous MI (important prognostic characteristic) and clinical site (i.e. hospital) (in order to negate inter-site differences). The trial was **double blind** and the 'endpoint classification committee' was also blinded to treatment allocation.

The primary **outcome** of the study was total mortality (i.e. 'counting the bodies', this was important as earlier studies had suggested that there may be an increase in sudden deaths in patients taking cholesterol-lowering agents). The secondary outcome was major coronary events and tertiary end-points including hospital admissions for acute CHD and the incidence of revascularization procedures. **Follow-up** procedures etc. were identical for both groups and median follow up was 5.4 years (range 4.9–6.3). All data were analyzed on an **intention-to-treat** basis, thus reflecting clinical practice. **Continuous data analysis** was performed and the trial was stopped early on the basis of the interim analysis showing that the study had achieved statistical significance that simvastatin was effective. The study did include two prospectively specified **subgroup analyses** (females and patients aged 60 or older) but the authors did recognize that these analyses 'had less statistical power'.

This study demonstrated significant reduction in all cause mortality:

11.5% in placebo group
8.2% in simvastatin group

Relative risk reduction (RRR) ~29%
Absolute risk reduction (ARR) ~3.3%
Numbers needed to treat (NNT) ~30

i.e. 30 patients with CHD and serum cholesterol in the range of 5.5–8.0 mmol/l need to be treated with simvastatin (20 mg) for 5.4 years to save one life. Adverse events were minor and similar in both groups.

This trial is worth reading as it is a good example of a well-conducted RCT and the answers to the 'quality control questions' stated above are all yes, except there is no confirmation (but it is implied) that no patients were lost to follow up.

Further reading

Collins R, Macmahon S. Reliable assessment of the effects of treatment on mortality and major morbidity, I: clinical trials. *Lancet* 2001; **357**: 373–380.
Guyatt GH, Sackett DL, Cook DJ. Users guide to the medical literature. II. How to use an article about therapy or prevention. B. What were the results and will they help me in caring for my patients? Evidence-Based Medicine Working Group. *JAMA* 1994; **271**(1): 59–63.

Related topics of interest

Outcome measures (p. 7); Critical appraisal (p. 70); Risk reduction and the number needed to treat (NNT) (p. 83); Bias and confounders (p. 101); Intention to treat (p. 105); Subgroup analysis (p. 117).

'OTHER' TRIALS FOR COMPARISON OF INTERVENTIONS

Dermot P.B. McGovern

Randomized controlled trials (RCTs) remain the gold standard for the comparison of interventions, however there are plenty of trials of other design comparing interventions published in the literature. These studies are often cheaper and easier to perform but come with disadvantages peculiar to each study design as discussed below.

Comparisons across time and place

The 'comparison across time' design uses historical control groups (who did not receive the experimental therapy) for comparison with current experimental groups. The fundamental problem with this concept is that the investigators have no 'control' over the control group. Ideally the control group should be treated identically to the experimental group with the exception of the experimental therapy. There is no doubt that over a period of time a number of other factors influencing outcome (personnel, social conditions, surgical techniques, other drugs) will also have changed. Hopefully, as time passes, through a host of medical advances, outcomes will improve and it is almost inevitable that studies that use historical controls will show benefit for the experimental therapy. This phenomenon was clearly demonstrated in a study comparing the results of RCTs and trials in which historical controls were used; approximately 80% of trials in which historical controls had been used showed a benefit for the intervention compared to a benefit in only 20% of RCTs. Most of this 'benefit' occurred as a result of the poor outcomes observed in the historical controls (see Further reading).

The Government's current vogue for 'league tables' of mortality rates for surgical procedures across hospitals is a good example of a comparison across places. These tables have rightly been criticized as presenting 'crude' data that do not allow for differences in important prognostic factors such as age and co-morbidity of patients etc. 'Respectable journals' would probably not consider studies of this design for publication yet they received significant copy in the non-medical press often without accompanying commentaries explaining the potential flaws in the data.

n = 1 trials

One of the valid criticisms of the EBM 'movement' is that it struggles to translate the results of large-scale trials into meaningful messages for dealing with individual patients. One more recent trial methodology that has been advocated to help overcome this is the $n = 1$ trial. This approach introduces a structure and more scientific rigour to the traditional trial and error ('suck it and see'!) trial of therapy. Traditionally a doctor would prescribe a medication and see the patient a few weeks later to assess response. If the patient's symptoms had improved then the treatment would continue, if not another one would be tried. Wearing a critical appraisal hat it is not difficult to see methodological flaws in this practice (unblinded, no control etc.). The $n = 1$ trial approach involves a patient being given one or another treatment (or placebo) in a random order and both patient and doctor being blinded to the nature of treatment (this would normally necessitate the help of an interested pharmacist). Each treatment period would last a specified length of time before the patient moved onto the next treatment. The patient would keep a diary of his or her symptoms and if possible use a validated questionnaire to monitor drug efficacy. At the end of the trial the drug regimens are un-blinded and the outcomes compared.

The ideal setting for this type of trial should include a helpful pharmacist, a willing patient with a chronic condition and a drug that acts quickly and does not have a long 'washout' period. An example of this would be a trial of different analgesics in a patient with painful osteoarthritis using validated pain scoring systems to judge the efficacy of the treatments. As in any trial it would be important to consider the adverse drug-related events in addition to the potential benefits.

This type of trial may be of use when the doctor cannot find evidence to answer a particular clinical question (because the trial has not been done) or is faced with a patient who would not meet the inclusion/exclusion criteria of the key study that may have answered the clinical question. It could be argued that this type of trial is the most sound of all trial methodologies and is probably the trial which produces data most applicable to the individual patient.

Uncontrolled trials

These could be considered as a less extreme version of a trial with historical controls. They are also known as 'before and after' trials as they evaluate outcomes before and after an intervention has been introduced and assume that any difference in the observed outcomes is due solely to the intervention itself. This is a dangerous assumption as there are often many other factors that change over a period of time that can influence outcomes (see Historical controls, above) and many diseases have unpredictable courses, i.e. symptoms may settle spontaneously following the intervention and thus a useless treatment may appear effective. A control group will 'correct' for this variability in disease activity and also for the effect of placebo and change in behaviour resulting from being in a trial (Hawthorne effect). One particular failing of some uncontrolled trials is that the investigators often don't think about starting a trial until the intervention has been introduced. They therefore, collect the post-intervention data prospectively (when all involved are usually aware of the study and may therefore modify their behaviour – another example of the Hawthorne effect) and are forced to collect the pre-intervention data retrospectively. This difference in data collection methods is clearly a potential source of bias.

Another type of uncontrolled study is the study whereby authors present a cohort of patients exposed to a particular intervention reporting what percentage have responded and how many have had adverse events. This type of study, again, cannot make allowances for variable disease activity, the effect of placebo or the Hawthorne effect. They can however answer the patient's question of 'What are my chances of being cured/going into remission etc. if I take this treatment?'. Of course this will not provide information to answer the query regarding the chance of cure/remission if the patient takes nothing. These studies usually consist of data collected retrospectively and are often presented as 'The St Elsewhere Hospital experience of.........'.

Non-random allocation trials

Bias is a significant problem with non-randomized trials in which the investigator (usually a doctor) decides which of the experimental treatments each individual patient should have. The investigator will have his/her own views as to which of the treatments is better and may (subconsciously) allocate patients with better prognoses to their 'favoured' treatment. They may also allocate patients they like to the perceived better treatment and 'work harder' for these patients. Non-random allocation inevitably means that the trial will not be blinded thereby introducing another potential source of bias.

Crossover trials

These should be considered a variation of the RCT in which the subjects on completing one of the trial therapies will receive another. Similar 'rules' apply to crossover trials with regard to blinding, randomization, etc. The great advantage of these trials is that fewer participants are needed as they all receive more than one therapy. It is important however to be sure that the therapies have a short 'carryover' period and that there is a suitably long enough 'washout' period between therapies, thus avoiding the effect (good or bad) of trial therapies continuing and influencing the outcome of the comparison therapy following crossover. A diagrammatic representation of a crossover trial is shown in Figure 1.

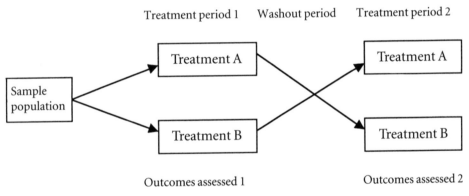

Figure 1. Diagrammatic representation of a crossover trial.

Example (Prophylactic treatment of migraine with angiotensin converting enzyme inhibitor (lisinopril): randomised, placebo controlled, crossover study. *BMJ* 2001; 322: 19–22)

This study enrolled 60 patients with migraine (2–6 episodes a month) and randomly allocated them to receive lisinopril for 12 weeks (10 mg for 1 week and 20 mg for 11 weeks), followed by a 2-week washout period, followed by 12 weeks of placebo (1 tablet for 1 week and 2 tablets for 11 weeks). Thirty patients followed this regimen and 30 patients received placebo first followed by lisinopril. The main outcome measures were number of hours with headache, number of days with headache and number of days with migraine.

The authors present the data on a completed therapy basis (47 patients) showing significant improvement in all the main outcomes in the lisinopril 'group'. On an 'intention to treat basis' of 55 patients (its not entirely clear what happened to the other five patients) there was a significant relative risk reduction for hours with headache (15% (95% CI 0 to 30%)), days with headache (16% (95% CI 5 to 27%)) and days with migraine (22% (95% CI 11 to 33%)). The pooled adverse events (no adverse events versus at least one symptom) showed a trend towards an increase with lisinopril ($p = 0.07$). The authors conclude that lisinopril has a place in migraine prophylaxis.

Further reading

Sachs H, Chalmers TC, Smith H. Randomized versus historical controls for clinical trials. *Am J Med* 1982; **72:** 233–240.

Related topics of interest

Randomized controlled trials (p. 25); Bias and confounders (p. 101).

COHORT STUDIES

Dermot P.B. McGovern

Case–control and cohort studies are analytical studies used to demonstrate associations between suspected causes and disease. Whilst there are important differences between the two types of study, many of the rules regarding design and interpretation of the results of the studies are applicable to both.

Aim

Cohort studies are observational studies designed to investigate the aetiology of diseases or outcomes. The aim of such studies is to investigate the link between a hypothetical cause and a defined outcome.

Design

Cohort studies originate with a hypothesis that the outcome (a disease) is caused by exposure to an event (risk factor). Subjects exposed to the suspected risk factor (cohort) and a similar group that have not been exposed (control) are identified. The two groups are followed prospectively over a period of time (usually a number of years) to identify the incidence of the outcome in both groups. These results are then analyzed to determine if the group exposed to the risk factor has a higher incidence of disease than those not exposed (see later). The design of a cohort study is summarized diagrammatically in Figure 1.

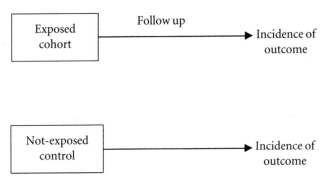

Figure 1. Diagrammatic representation of cohort studies.

Cohort studies are usually prospective but they can be performed retrospectively if there is a clearly documented point of first exposure. Occupational records have been successfully used in this way.

When identifying subjects for control and cohort groups investigators should remember that follow up will normally last a number of years and hence the study populations should be as cooperative, contactable and non-migratory as possible. Additional care should be taken in accumulating the control population as it is essential that apart from the risk factor under investigation both groups should be equally susceptible to the disease in question i.e. the groups should be well matched. If the groups are not matched then the results of the study should be treated with caution. Matching helps avoid **confounding variables** – variables that can independently affect (both increase and decrease) the risk and are associated with the hypothetical cause. For example a cohort study may demonstrate that men who drink excess alcohol have an increased risk of developing lung cancer. This is not a causal relationship and the confounding variable is smoking as men who drink more alcohol also smoke more. The effect of confounding variables can be corrected for using the **Mantel–Haenszel equation** (see case–control studies). The above example also highlights the very important point that any association demonstrated by a cohort (or case–control) study does not *prove* a causal relationship.

Prior to undertaking a cohort study investigators should seek statistical advice regarding the number of subjects needed in each group. This will depend on predicted attributable risk (see later) and the length of follow up proposed.

Disadvantages of cohort studies
- Time consuming and costly (unless the outcome has a high incidence and short latent period).
- Long studies inevitably increase the drop-out rates.
- Cohort studies are not useful investigations for rare diseases as large numbers of subjects are required.

Advantages of cohort studies
- The prospective design of the 'standard' cohort study provides an opportunity for accurate data collection that is not normally available from retrospective studies.
- The incidence, relative risk and attributable risk can be calculated from the results.
- An estimate of the time from exposure to disease development is possible.
- Occasionally cohort studies can be performed retrospectively and can thus be cheaper and less time consuming.

Results

If the data are qualitative then it is standard practice to present the data as a '2 by 2' table as shown below. Quantitative data will require grouping or correlation calculations in order to demonstrate associations.

	Affected	Unaffected	Total	Risk
Exposed	a	b	N_1	$a/N_1 = r_e$
Unexposed	c	d	N_0	$c/N_0 = r_o$
Total	M_1	M_0	T	

The **Relative risk** $(RR) = r_e / r_o$.
The **Odds ratio** $(OR) = ad / bc$.
The **Attributable risk** $= r_e - r_o$.

To determine whether a result is statistically significant it is standard practice to perform a chi-squared (χ^2) test to calculate a P value and confidence limits (the significance and use of P values, confidence limits, relative risks and odds ratios are covered in more detail elsewhere in this book).

Attributable risk is the absolute amount of the outcome (disease) that is associated with the exposure. Attributable is a poor description as it implies causation, which is not necessarily the case. If the study conclusion is that there is a causative relationship then attributable risks can help prioritize interventions that will have the most impact on preventing the outcome.

If the results do demonstrate an increased risk for one of the groups a number of questions still need to be addressed:

- Has the result occurred by chance? Evaluation of the statistical analysis will help exclude this.
- Has the result occurred as a consequence of bias? **Ascertainment bias** occurs when data are collected in different ways in the control and cohort groups. **Selection bias** can occur when subjects (from either group) are excluded because they have an association with the suspected cause.
- If the association is real is it a cause and effect relationship? Some authorities have said causation is more likely if:
  1. There is a strong association.
  2. The association is graded (i. e. there is a dose–response relationship).
  3. The association is independent and standardization of the data (negating the effects of confounding variables) does not abolish the relationship.
  4. The association is demonstrated in more than one study and population.
  5. The association makes sense.

Quality control questions for cohort studies

Note that these are similar to those for case–control studies

1. Were the groups similar apart from the exposure under question?
2. Were the data on outcomes collected identically in both groups?
3. Is there a dose–response effect?
4. Does the relationship make biological and chronological sense?
5. How strong is the association and how precise is the estimate?
6. Is the risk of sufficient magnitude that exposure should be abolished?

Example (Mortality in relation to smoking: 20 years' observations on male British doctors. *BMJ* 1976; 2: 1525–1536)

This study by Doll and Peto is probably one of the most famous cohort studies of all time. In 1951 they sent questionnaires to all doctors (this study only reports the results from the male doctors) on the British medical register asking about their smoking habits. A total of 34 440 (69%) responded and were included in their trial. Cause of mortality in trial participants was observed from 1951 to 1971. Additional information about change in smoking habits was obtained through follow-up questionnaires. At the end of the study (1971) 10 072 subjects had died, 24 265 were definitely alive and 103 (0.3%) had been lost to follow up.

Over the 20-year period cigarette smoking had reduced from, on average, 9.1 to 3.6 cigarettes per day per doctor. The mortality results for lung cancer and ischaemic heart disease are shown in Table 1.

Table 1. The annual death rate per 100000 men from lung cancer and ischaemic heart disease for smokers and non-smokers

	Annual death rate per 100000 men, standardized for age	
	Lung cancer	Ischaemic heart disease
Non-smokers	10	413
Cigarettes smokers		
Overall	140	669
1–14/day	78	608
15–24	127	652
> 25	251	792

It can be seen from these figures that increased rates of death from lung cancer and ischaemic heart disease (IHD) are associated with heavier smoking. Since these figures are rates/100000/year they all have common denominators and so the relative risk for lung cancer in smokers versus non-smokers is 140/10 = 14.

- RR for lung cancer in smokers of >25 cigarettes/day versus non-smokers is 251/10 = 25.1.
- RR for IHD in smokers versus non-smokers = 669/413 ~ 1.62.

Thus it can be seen that the relative risk for lung cancer is considerably higher than that for IHD in smokers. However these are relative values and the public health effect of abolishing smoking totally can be better judged by viewing the attributable risk:

- Attributable risk for smoking in lung cancer = 140 – 10 = 130/100000/year.
- Attributable risk for smoking in IHD = 669 – 413 = 256/100000/year.

Thus despite the higher relative risk for lung cancer, smoking abolition would have a greater overall impact on IHD as it is a more common disease.

This study could be criticized for not quoting confidence intervals and P values but this was not normal practice at this time. This is a seminal paper and well worth a read.

Further reading

Levine M, Walter SD, Lee H *et al*. User's guides to the medical literature: IV. How to use an article about harm. *JAMA* 1994; **271**: 1615–1619.

Related topics of interest

CASE–CONTROL STUDIES

Dermot P.B. McGovern

Case–control and cohort studies are analytical studies used to demonstrate associations between suspected causes and disease. Whilst there are important differences between the two types of study, many of the rules regarding design and interpretation of the studies are applicable to both.

Aim

Like cohort studies, case–control studies are analytical epidemiological studies whose aim is to investigate the association between disease and suspected causes.

Design

In case–control studies people with an outcome (disease) are identified and **then** their medical and social history is examined retrospectively in an attempt to identify exposure to potential risk factors. A matched control group of people/patients (free from the disease) are also identified and data collected from them in an identical fashion. The two sets of data are compared to determine whether the disease group was exposed in significantly higher numbers to the suspected risk factors than the control group. The design of a case–control study is summarized diagrammatically in Figure 1.

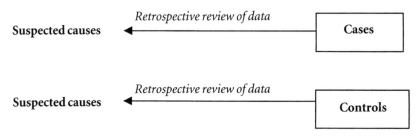

Figure 1. Diagrammatic representation of case–control study.

Case–control studies can also be used to provide evidence ascertaining whether medical interventions have been effective or not. For example, the history of attendance for cervical cancer screening in women who have died of cervical cancer (cases) could be compared with age-matched women who had not died of cervical cancer (controls). A significantly higher uptake in women who had not died of cancer would suggest that this form of screening is effective (though it is worth remembering that people who are health conscious (and thus less likely to develop cancer) are more likely to attend for screening).

When designing a case–control study it is important to tightly define what constitutes a 'case'. Cases can be incidence cases (newly diagnosed) or prevalent cases (existing cases). The former on the whole provide better data as they will have improved recall (from more recent events) and probably better records.

Choosing controls for a case–control study can also be difficult and it is important to ensure:

- That controls do not have the disease/outcome being investigated in the study (if a number of them do then this will tend to bias the results towards the null hypothesis).
- That it is possible to collect data from the controls in exactly the same way as from the cases (avoiding ascertainment bias).
- That controls should be a representative sample of the eligible population (who are free of the disease in question).

A number of sources are commonly used to identify appropriate controls including: other patients (in-patients, patients from other clinics or patients from the same primary care practice), relatives, neighbours or simply 'the general population'. Relatives may be a good source of controls as they are genetically similar to the cases and also often have similar environments.

It is not always possible to totally exclude confounding factors from influencing the results of a case–control (or a cohort) study. There are a number of methods available to help overcome this and probably the most commonly used involves stratification of the data into strata defined by the levels of exposure to the confounding factor. Odds ratios can be calculated for each stratum and using the **Mantel–Haenszel equation** it is possible to produce a weighted average of the odds ratios from the different strata. This odds ratio is an estimate of the unconfounded odds ratio.

 Confounders for

Disadvantages of case–control study

- It is not possible to calculate the true incidence and relative risk. The results should be expressed as odds ratios.
- The study design inevitably means that data are collected retrospectively and hence the information may not be available or may be of poor quality.

Advantages of case–control study

- These studies are relatively quick and cheap to perform.
- Case–control studies are useful for investigating rare diseases.
- Case–control studies can be used to evaluate interventions.

Results

In a similar way to cohort studies the results of case–control study can be expressed as a '2 × 2' table (see below) if the data are qualitative (if the disease and suspected cause can be recorded as present or absent). If the data are quantitative (e.g. haemoglobin concentration or systolic blood pressure) then interpretation will either require grouping of data or demonstration of a correlation. This also applies to cohort studies.

	Affected (cases)	Unaffected (controls)
Exposed	a	b
Unexposed	c	d

$$\text{Odds ratio (OR)} = a/b/c/d = \frac{a\,d}{b\,c}$$

To determine whether a result is statistically significant it is standard practice to perform a chi-squared (χ^2) test to calculate a P value and confidence limits.

Statistically significant results by themselves are not enough to conclude that there is a causative link between the exposure and the outcome. A number of questions still need to be answered (see under cohort study) before this conclusion can be reached.

Quality control questions for case–control studies

1. Were the groups similar apart from the exposure under question?
2. Were the data on outcomes collected identically in both groups?
3. Is there a dose–response effect?
4. Does the relationship make biological and chronological sense?
5. How strong is the association and how precise is the estimate?
6. Is the risk of sufficient magnitude that exposure should be abolished?

Example (Symptomatic gastroesophageal reflux as a risk factor for esophageal adenocarcinoma. *New England Journal of Medicine* 1999; 340: 825–831)

This large Swedish case–control study examined the association between gastro-oesophageal reflux and oesophageal adenocarcinoma. They identified 189 patients with oesophageal adenocarcinoma and selected 820 age- and sex-matched controls from the Swedish population. The data regarding symptoms of heartburn were collected from the two groups in a similar fashion. The results are summarized in Table 1.

Table 1. Data from example study investigating the association between gastro-oesophageal reflux and oesophageal adenocarcinoma

	Oesophageal adenocarcinoma (cases)	General population (controls)
Heartburn, regurgitation or both at least once a week	113 (a)	135 (b)
No heartburn etc.	76 (c)	685 (d)

$$\text{Odds ratio} = a/b/c/d = \frac{a\,d}{b\,c} = \frac{113 \times 685}{76 \times 135} = 7.5$$

(Note in the paper they quote adjusted odds ratios as well as 95% confidence intervals – odds ratio of 7.7 [5.3–11.4].)

The authors also demonstrated that the more frequent, the more severe and the longer lasting the symptoms of reflux the greater the risk of developing oesophageal adenocarcinoma (dose–response relationship) with odds ratios up to 43.5 (95% C.I. 18.3–103.5). The authors conclude that 'there is a strong and probable causal relation between gastro-oesophageal reflux and oesophageal adenocarcinoma'. It is well worth reading this well conducted trial as a good example of a case–control study.

Further reading

Levine M, Walter SD, Lee H *et al.* User's guides to the medical literature: IV. How to use an article about harm. *Journal of the American Medical Association* 1994; **271:** 1615–1619.

Related topics of interest

Cohort studies (p. 33); Statistical methods (p. 73); The *P* value (p. 77); Relative risk, relative risk reduction and odds ratio (p. 79); Confidence intervals (p. 87).

CROSS-SECTIONAL (PREVALENCE) SURVEYS

Dermot P.B. McGovern

Cross-sectional studies are descriptive studies in which a sample population's status is determined for the presence or absence of exposure and disease *at the same time*. These surveys take a 'snapshot' of the population and thus detect the presence of disease at a point in time (prevalence) as opposed to the frequency of onset of the disease (incidence). Figure 1 is a diagrammatic representation of a cross-sectional survey.

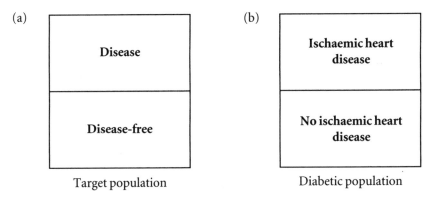

Figure 1. Diagrammatic representation of a cross-sectional survey (a) and a theoretical example examining the prevalence of ischaemic heart disease in a diabetic population (b).

Basic principles

In principle these surveys should begin with a complete list of the target population from which a randomly selected sample population is chosen. Data, usually from questionnaires or interviews, are obtained about individuals in the sample population regarding their current status. Data can be collected about any factors that influence health status including age, sex, ethnicity, smoking status, occupation etc. No group is selected as a control group but 'internal' comparisons are possible (e.g. men versus women from within the group).

Role of cross-sectional surveys

- The data can be used to determine a relationship between exposure and disease, i.e. a survey may show that there is a higher incidence of ischaemic heart disease (IHD) in diabetic patients than in non-diabetics. However there is no temporal relationship in these studies and it is impossible to distinguish between cause and effect, i.e. does diabetes cause IHD or are people with IHD more likely to develop diabetes. For this reason surveys such as this can be regarded as hypothesis-generating rather than hypothesis-testing. There is one exception to this rule and that is where disease is found to be associated with a 'fixed' factor such as race, sex, blood group etc. a situation which makes hypothesis 'proving' much easier.

- These types of studies have been used to demonstrate the prevalence of diseases in specified occupations such as respiratory disease in rubber factory workers.

- Governments may make use of large-scale cross-sectional studies, for example The Health Interview Survey (HIS) from the United States in which over 100 000 'representative people' are interviewed about disease prevalence, healthcare use, days off work sick, smoking status, age, ethnicity, socio-economic status etc. The government use these data to assist in the planning of future provision of healthcare.

Potential problems

Like any other study cross-sectional surveys are prone to bias and particular problems to watch out for include:

- **Left censorship,** the phenomenon where people in the defined population may have had the disease in question but (as the study measures prevalence) may not be recorded as they have died, migrated or even fully recovered. For example a cross-sectional survey may show that the prevalence of IHD is higher in Caucasians than Afro-Caribbeans. This however ignores the fact that 'Afro-Caribbean IHD' may be more severe and these people may die quicker. So, in spite of the fact that the incidence may be higher and the disease more severe in Afro-Caribbeans, a cross-sectional survey may give the impression that IHD is a much greater problem in Caucasians.

- People who respond to health surveys are likely to have different characteristics to those who do not. Poor responders include males, those at extremes of age and those of low socio-economic class. One example of a biased survey was the study to detect the prevalence of diabetes within a population. The results showed a particularly high prevalence but it became apparent that the population had self-selected as a very high percentage of those who attended were more likely to have had symptoms of thirst etc. or had a family history of diabetes.

- The problem of cause and effect is particularly pertinent to cross-sectional surveys given the 'snapshot' type of data they produce.

Example (Cross sectional study of differences in coronary artery calcification by socio-economic status. *BMJ* 2000; 321: 1262–1263)

This study used electron beam computed tomography to quantify coronary artery calcification (a validated measure of coronary plaque volume) in 149 30–40-year-old people. The aim of the study was to determine a relationship between coronary artery calcification and socio-economic status. The participants were randomly sampled from two general practices (but there was no mention of how many people declined to take part in the study) and social class was determined by present occupation using the Registrar General's classification and whether they were in full-time education at the age of 19. Being in the manual social class was associated with a higher prevalence of calcification with an odds ratio of 2.3 (95% CI 1.3 to 5.2, $P = 0.04$) and so was having left full time education by 19 years of age, odds ratio of 2.8 (95% CI 1.2 to 6.3, $P = 0.01$). Adjusting for other risk factors of coronary artery disease only slightly altered the odds ratio although the statistical significance was reduced. It is of course possible (but unlikely) that coronary artery disease is more aggressive in higher socio-economic groups (through left censorship), which could also explain these results. These results have generated the hypothesis that lower socio-economic status is an independent risk factor for coronary artery disease and this now needs to be confirmed (hypothesis testing) by observational studies (cohort and case–control studies).

Related topic of interest

Determining causation (p. 4).

CASE REPORTS AND CASE SERIES

Marcel Levi

A rough search in the MEDLINE database from 1997 until 2000 reveals that up to about 25% of published papers in clinical journals are case reports or case series. Hence, this most classical form of medical reporting remains popular. A case report describes a characteristic or maybe uncharacteristic medical history of a patient, usually with a relatively rare disorder or remarkable clinical course. The purpose of this report is to communicate a particular clinical presentation, diagnosis or treatment to the medical community, illustrated by the history of the selected patient. A case series is essentially the same, but in this type of publication more than one patient is demonstrated. In fact, case reports and case series cannot be regarded as forms of medical research, but merely reflect the personal experience of the authors. Case reports and case series are conventionally regarded as one of the lowest forms of clinical evidence based on a number of considerations that are outlined below. However, these types of medical publications may play a role and have some merit (see later).

Limited value of case reports and case series

Example: You have just received notification that your son is due for his measles, mumps and rubella (MMR) vaccination. He is fit and healthy and has received all of his vaccinations to date with no ill effects. You read in the newspaper that a case series from London has shown a link between MMR and autism. However when you read the original paper (*Lancet* 1998; **351:** 637–641) you realize that the report concerned 12 children with loss of skills plus gastrointestinal disease, associated (by the parents or a physician) in eight cases with MMR vaccination. Vaccination rates in the general population at the time were around 90+% so (as the authors admitted) no link could be proven.

This example shows that case reports and case-series are often not very helpful. It is unfortunate for the children involved that they developed autism but there is little evidence that MMR vaccination was involved. In fact, it may well be that we are not looking at an adverse effect of MMR vaccination, but simply the natural history of autism in these particular cases resulting in a temporal link. Moreover, the case-series does not make us aware of the potential harm caused by not vaccinating children with MMR. Since there is no control group the true existence of a link cannot be confirmed nor can the magnitude of any effect be estimated. Case-reports and case-series typically report the history and outcomes from selected patients, hence, the applicability to patients in general (i.e. your next patient) is unclear (your son does not have inflammatory bowel disease). Apart from these considerations, case-series and case-reports may suffer from serious publication bias. Understandably interesting new findings or treatment options generate more interest from reviewers and journal editors, and may thus be more likely to be accepted for publication.

Promising or surprising results in case-report and case-series are often premature and there are many examples of initial findings that could not be corroborated in sound controlled clinical trials. Hence, conclusions from these reports should be interpreted with maximal caution. As far as MMR goes, the published literature since Wakefield's original report has been almost totally negative.

Merit of case reports and case series

Example: In 1997 the *New England Journal of Medicine* published a report on a series of 24 previously healthy and relatively young women, who developed valvular heart disease. Importantly, all these women had started to use fenfluramine-phentermine as weight-losing (appetite-depressing) agents about 1 year prior to the manifestation of their heart disease. The authors of this report concluded that their findings suggest concern that this drug causes serious valvular heart disease.

This second example illustrates the strength of case reports and case series. These increasingly widely used, appetite-depressant agents appeared to cause a serious adverse effect. Since the chance of getting this complication is relatively rare, a controlled clinical trial would probably not have had the power to detect this complication. In such a situation, a case report or a case series may be very helpful to quickly report a potential hazard or adverse effect of therapy. Obviously, such an observation deserves further confirmation, for example in a case–control study. In the case of the example, later studies indeed showed a highly elevated risk of developing valvular heart disease in woman taking these agents. Hence, case reports and case series may serve as early indicators of novel developments, risks, and diagnostic or therapeutic options but their significance is limited to the provocation and stimulation of scientifically more powerful investigations, such as case–control studies or prospective controlled trials. In other words case reports and case series should be regarded as hypothesis-generating, but not hypothesis-proving types of reports.

Further reading

Connolly HM *et al.* Valvular heart disease associated with fenfluramine-phentermine. *N Engl J Med* 1997; **337:** 581–588.

Goringe AP *et al.* Glutamine and vitamin E in the treatment of veno-occlusive disease following high-dose chemotherapy. *Bone Marrow Transpl* 1998; **21:** 829–832.

QUALITATIVE RESEARCH

William S.M. Summerskill

Qualitative research explains social interactions, and provides insight to questions of 'how?' and 'why?'. In contrast to quantitative research, which sets out to challenge an existing hypothesis, qualitative research is hypothesis-generating. Just as quantitative research employs different trial designs to answer different questions, qualitative research also uses a variety of approaches. Qualitative studies have a special role in evidence-based medicine. Understanding patient and practitioner attitudes and behaviour, allows evidence to be applied in the most effective manner.

Paradigms

Qualitative approaches arise from sociological investigations and reflect different, occasionally competing, schools of sociological thought. These perspectives influence research design and determine how observations will be interpreted. Important considerations are the concept of truth being relative, rather than absolute, and the concept of the investigator as participant in research.

Like quantitative studies, the outcome reflects the study population. Whereas this 'truth' will be valid for the study group, it is rarely *generalizable*. Instead, robust qualitative findings may be *transferable* to different settings.

Participation in research affects behaviour (the Hawthorne effect). Qualitative data can involve interviews in which the behaviour of both subject and researcher influence outcomes. This interaction is embraced by qualitative research as part of the investigative process. Objectivity is maintained through *reflexivity*, a process of self-awareness (often documented in a diary by the researcher) and used to identify and understand sources of bias.

Qualitative approaches

The choice of study design is determined by the research question. Types of study are listed below in increasing size, from the individual, to the group, to the culture.

Phenomenology describes individuals' experiences related to a specific event, in order to understand the essence of that event. Numbers involved are small (usually less than 10) as data collection involves in-depth interviews to explore individuals' experiences and reflections on the phenomenon. Interpretation should distinguish between the participant's subjective narrative and the researcher's objective findings.

Grounded theory uses a group's experience to construct a theory of behaviour 'grounded' in observations. Observations on 20–30 individuals are coded according to themes and then integrated to create an inductive description. The process is characterized by the *constant comparative method* in which new findings are compared with the evolving theory and used to guide the ongoing research. The investigator(s) must have a broad understanding of the study situation, without any specific bias.

Action (participatory) research involves a co-operative approach between researcher and subjects (co-researchers). Opportunities are identified and then incorporated into an agreed action to promote change. A cyclical approach helps to reinforce previous changes and consider new directions.

Ethnography, the study of culture, defines beliefs and behaviour within a population sharing a common identity. The identity could be demographic, illness or behavioural. Subject numbers vary from 15 upwards. Through observation from within the study culture's own environment, the researcher strives to achieve the '*emic*' or 'insider's view' of that culture. Observations should not be contaminated as a result of his/her own actions or questions, and should include minority views within the culture. The basis for any interpretation of beliefs must be explicit.

Qualitative tools

1. ***Sampling*** in qualitative research is not random. As the numbers involved are small and the time investment is large, participants are selected on their ability to inform the process, rather than their representativeness of society as a whole.

- **Critical case sampling** involves the selection of individuals who will provide the greatest quality of information.
- **Theoretical sampling** is guided by emerging findings in grounded theory to identify subjects for further data collection. An important process for assuring that data are complete and robust.
- **Extreme sampling** purposefully seeks individuals at the extremes of the phenomenon under study. This adds breadth to the data and can identify 'deviant cases' for testing hypotheses.
- **Stratified sampling** uses pre-specified criteria to create categories of interest from which subjects are recruited. This approach enhances generalizability.
- **Snowball sampling** identifies key individuals through whom other subjects are contacted as a result of their relationship to that individual. This is a useful method to recruit specific populations which might otherwise be difficult to interest. Success is dependent upon the initial individuals and a clear understanding of the contact network.
- **Convenience sampling** describes the use of a population who were willing to participate, but do not necessarily fulfil any of the above criteria. Convenience samples are the least desirable population to study as their data may be variable in quality or biased by the relationship with the investigator that resulted in their inclusion.

2. ***Data collection*** can involve artefacts, documents, interviews or any combination of these. The reason for choosing a specific data type should be explicit.

- **Interviews** are the commonest source of data. Interviews can be informal, guided or structured. More formal interviews ensure that specific topics are included, but lack flexibility to explore other issues. Interviews can be recorded by observer notes or electronically. Electronic recording provides an accurate record of conversation, but may require observer notes to describe non-verbal interactions. The more intrusive the recording equipment (such as a video camera), the greater the risk of distracting the participant. The number of interviewers and their training will affect data collection. The method of data recording and transcription should be stated, along with any techniques used to capture non-verbal details.

- **Semi-structured interviews** involve prepared open-ended questions, but allow flexibility to explore issues in greater detail or to consider unexpected topics. Details about the origin of the instrument are important, and a copy of the interview schedule (sometimes available on journal websites) helps to explain the findings. Individual interviews are time-consuming, but yield large amounts of data.
- **Focus groups** involve 8–15 participants and a facilitator 'focusing' on the topic of interest. They can be a time-efficient way to collect information. Focus groups offer the benefit of encouraging discussions between individuals, and thereby exploring subjects that might not have arisen in individual sessions. One potential disadvantage is domination by some participants and reluctance of other participants to express contradictory opinions. Focus groups are inappropriate for some personal subjects.
- **Delphi technique** allows individuals to concentrate on issues rather than personalities. Anonymous responses are circulated among the participants in a repeated cycle of comment and review until a consensus is achieved. This is useful for geographically separated participants as it can be accomplished by post or e-mail.
- **Card (pile) sorting** involves a pile of cards, which subjects arrange according to their order of preference. The cards may contain illustrations or statements, and can also be used as props for further discussion. The process clarifies attitudes and decision-making processes, but the pre-determined nature of the cards can limit the information gained.
- **Feedback sessions** allow participants to comment on study findings (respondent validation). Corroboration of findings is important, and often leads to further insights from participants. Rejection of the findings allows participants to re-focus the study.

3. Triangulation describes the navigational technique of using separate measurements to establish a position. Similarly, qualitative studies will use complementary approaches to produce separate perspectives of a phenomenon, resulting in a clearer understanding of that phenomenon.

Interpretation

The fundamental principles of critical appraisal apply to any qualitative paper. Is the research designed appropriately and conducted rigorously with absence of bias? Are the findings considered carefully, and the conclusions substantiated?

The research question should be clearly formulated, with an appropriate choice of trial design. Background information should describe the reason for the research and the investigators' perspective. It need not include a literature review, since some qualitative researchers argue that a literature review will introduce bias. However, if a literature review is included, expect the authors to have checked relevant sociological databases.

Methods, such as sampling, will be clearly described, referenced, and appropriate to the research question and population. A 'second reader' would be expected in any transcript analysis to confirm findings. The second reader should be an experienced qualitative researcher who identifies transcript themes independently. This provides a source of objectivity, so that an investigator's interpretation of statements is not influenced by his/her own bias. Qualitative computer software, such as *NUD*IST* or *ATLAS*, may be used as a data handling and retrieval tool. These programmes do not perform data analysis (other than searches), and do not imply greater credibility of findings.

Expect 'saturation', data collection that has continued until no new themes have been identified. The findings section should contain source material, such as quotes, which describe the results. Like appraising quantitative research, one is looking for consistent data. This is measured by 'depth' and 'richness' of findings. 'Deviant case analysis' seeks out contradictory examples to test any emerging theory. Reflexivity will describe the researcher's involvement and response to the study.

The discussion section should include alternative explanations for the findings. Having substantiated the conclusions, the paper ought to consider opportunities and limitations for transferability.

Example

To explore the experience of diabetes in a British Bangladeshi population, Greenhalgh *et al.* used critical case sampling to identify 44 subjects, 40 of whom participated (*BMJ* 1998; **316:** 978–983). Data were collected by semi-structured interviews, focus groups/feedback sessions, narratives and pile sorting. Four separate piles involved ranking the severity of diabetes *vs.* other diseases, the appropriateness of different foods for diabetics, healthy menus, and photographs to elicit desirable body size. Multiple methods provided triangulation. The respondents attributed diabetes to divine will, they viewed larger body size and sugar/fat containing foods as healthy, and exercise was considered as potentially weakening. Only qualitative research could illustrate such significant cultural attitudes, which complicate the management of diabetes in this population.

Further reading

Grbich C. *Qualitative Research in Health*. London: Sage, 1999.
Mays N, Pope C. Assessing Quality in Qualitative Research. *BMJ* 2000; **320:** 50–52.

Related topics of interest

Hierarchy of evidence (p. 13); Sources of information (p. 57); Sites of interest on the World Wide Web (p. 60); Search strategies for electronic databases (p. 63); Critical appraisal (p. 70).

SCREENING

Dermot P.B. McGovern

Screening is an intervention (history, examination or investigation) for the detection of previously unrecognized disease or disease risk factors in order to treat/modify the disease/risk factor thereby leading to an improved prognosis.

Rationale for screening

The fundamental principles underlying the process of screening are:

- The disease in question can be detected long before it is clinically apparent to the patient (i.e. before symptoms or signs would have developed resulting in the patient seeking medical advice).
- Disease detected at an earlier stage has, given appropriate treatment, a significantly better outlook than disease treated when symptoms become apparent.

EBM has a significant role to play in the whole debate regarding screening. Screening is an intervention similar to any other and is thus most appropriately evaluated using a randomized controlled trial (RCT). However because of the nature (long natural history) of many of the diseases thought suitable for screening and because the large majority of people screened in such trials will be free from disease these trials are inevitably expensive and require long follow-up times and large numbers of people. Therefore correlation studies and observational (case–control and) cohort studies have also been used to evaluate screening tests:

- Correlation studies could examine the relationship between disease rates (or disease fatality rates) and the frequency of screening for the disease within a population.
- Case–control studies could examine the frequency of screening in a group of patients with the disease and the frequency of screening in a matched control group (without the disease).
- Cohort studies could examine the fatality rate in those diagnosed at screening compared to those diagnosed following presentation with symptoms to assess whether there is a better prognosis in those diagnosed through screening.

It is important to remember that potential screening interventions should also be evaluated with regard to cost-effectiveness and their effect on the quality of people's lives.

Ethical issues

A number of important ethical issues regarding screening should always be addressed when considering the introduction of a screening test. In comparison to 'normal' medical practice the process of screening occurs as a result of the health care establishment approaching a healthy person (and not a patient with symptoms presenting themselves). In light of this any potential harmful effects of being entered into a screening programme must be seriously considered including:

- Potentially harmful investigations. Investigations that cause harm in healthy people e.g. colonoscopy with approximately a 1 in 1500 perforation rate would have to be viewed suspiciously in the screening context as the overall benefits of screening are already likely to be marginal.
- Potentially harmful treatments. For example screening, by ultrasound, for asymptomatic abdominal aortic aneurysms (AAA) in 50–60-year-old men; identification of an aneurysm would lead to an operation (otherwise there is no point in screening), which carries a significant mortality. This type of intervention would have to recognize that some of the men who died in the operating theatre may well have never had any problems with their AAA.
- Harm from being 'labelled' as having a positive result from the screening test. A positive result does not mean a definitive diagnosis and people with false positive results will usually undergo further investigations and even potentially harmful treatment. There is evidence from breast screening programmes that women who have abnormal mammograms but are then shown to be disease-free (false positives) suffer considerable anxiety even after being given the 'all clear'.
- Likewise a negative test does not definitively mean that the person does not have the disease and people may become complacent about worrying symptoms as a result of the 'reassurance' of a negative test.

The issue that positive screening tests do not necessarily mean disease and that negative tests do not necessarily mean disease-free is an extremely important issue regarding screening that health care professionals need to educate the general public about.

Which diseases are candidates for screening?

A number of well documented criteria need to be met before a disease should be considered for a screening programme including:

- Is the disease common and/or does it have serious consequences (morbidity and mortality)?
- Does the disease have a well-defined natural history? This enables the development of a screening test that can be used to identify the disease early in its natural history. Does this 'precursor' (identified at screening) definitively and inexorably develop into the disease?
- Does treatment earlier in the natural history of the disease lead to improved outcomes?
- Who in the population is at risk of the disease and will they attend for screening?
- Is there a test available that is safe, accurate and acceptable? Ideally the test should have high sensitivity and specificity and therefore a high likelihood ratio. It is worth remembering that as screening invariably means 'investigation' of healthy people the vast majority of them will not have the disease. Therefore the pre-test probabilities of any single one of the patients having the disease will be low. Thus in spite of high likelihood ratios the post-test probability is also likely

to be low (this is Bayes theorem and is discussed in more detail in the chapter on pre- and post test probabilities and likelihood ratios). This explains the rationale for identifying groups at higher risk for the disease (a process known as case finding) as this will increase the screening test's pre-test probability.

- Is there an effective and acceptable treatment for the disease if it can be diagnosed early?
- Can the health service infrastructure cope with the increased number of tests and 'treatments' that will inevitable result from a screening programme?
- Will the screening programme be cost-effective and could the money be better spent elsewhere?

Potential sources of bias in screening evaluation

Studies examining the effectiveness of screening programmes should undergo a quality evaluation in a similar way to other studies. The same principles apply as discussed in the chapters on observational studies and RCTs. However there are three sources of bias that are particularly pertinent to screening studies:

1. Lead time bias. This occurs when a screening test identifies a disease earlier in the course of the natural history. Early identification may not alter the prognosis but the person will know for longer that they have the condition. Examination of survival time will suggest longer survival for the screened patient than the patient who presents with symptoms but this will only be because the disease was identified earlier. Lead time bias is represented diagrammatically in Figure 1.

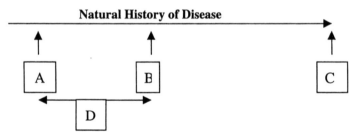

Figure 1. A diagrammatic representation of lead time bias of a fatal disease in a 'screened' patient and an 'unscreened' patient.
Arrow A – Patient 1 diagnosed by screening; Arrow B – Patient 2 presented with symptoms; Arrow C – Patient 1 and 2 both die of the disease; Arrow D represents the apparent improved length of survival (the lead time bias) that screening has provided.

2. Length bias. Screening is more likely to identify slowly progressive disease than aggressive disease and therefore an apparent benefit on length of survival through screening may be demonstrated as a result of this different case mixture.

3. Compliance bias. Compliant patients have better outcomes across the board than non-compliant ones. Therefore screening studies that make use of volunteers in their active group and non-volunteers in their control group may well exaggerate any beneficial effects of screening.

There are a number of well documented screening programmes in operation and Bandolier have compiled a screening black- (of unproven (cost)effectiveness) and white-list (of proven cost-effectiveness) of screening programmes in response to an article that appeared in *The Times* suggesting people should be seeking a whole variety of screening tests. The page on screening in Bandolier is well worth looking at (www.jr2.ox.ac.uk/Bandolier).

The whole debate about screening is controversial and a recent meta-analysis evaluating breast cancer screening highlights this (see Further reading). This review identified eight randomized trials (containing over 450000 women) but the authors argued that six of these contained significant flaws in terms of the randomization process. A sensitivity analysis was performed and this demonstrated that:

- When the results from the two 'good' trials were pooled and analyzed there was no significant benefit from deaths from breast cancer between screened and unscreened women (relative risk 1.04, 95% CI 0.85–1.25; number needed to screen – 10570, 95% CI 2138–1522).
- When the six 'bad' trials' results were pooled there was a more favourable result with a relative risk of 0.75 (95% CI 0.67–0.83; number needed to screen 661, 506–950).
- The overall pooled results (from all eight trials) did demonstrate a benefit from screening with a relative risk of 0.80 (95% CI 0.73–0.88; number needed to screen 1040, 755–1672).

The authors of this paper question the validity of the evidence showing the benefit of breast cancer screening. They also demonstrate that the higher the breast cancer death rate in the unscreened population (i.e. reflecting the underlying prevalence in the general population) the more likely the screening programme would show an overall benefit. Finally, they argued that the difference in breast cancer death rates between the primary studies was far greater than the difference resulting from screening. This review is worth reading as it not only highlights some of the problems of screening but also those of meta-analyses and the potential benefits of sensitivity analysis.

Further reading

Gotzsche PC and Olsen O. Is screening for breast cancer with mammography justifiable? *Lancet* 2000; **355:** 129–134.

Related topics of interest

Sensitivity and specificity (p. 90); Pre- and post-test probabilities (p. 000); Likelihood ratios (p. 92); Negative/positive predictive values (p. 96).

QUESTIONNAIRES

William S.M. Summerskill

Questionnaires provide valuable patient-based evidence. They can identify prognostic groups, assess interventions and monitor health status. Questionnaires can be either quantitative or qualitative. Quantitative instruments allow quicker analysis; qualitative surveys give richer data. Both methods can be combined. Instruments must have proven efficacy and be appropriate for the intended population.

Development

Questions should be derived from the concept being measured (e.g. patient satisfaction, functional impairment from rheumatoid arthritis). Interviews and focus groups identify core themes to define the concept.

Statements (questions) are derived from the themes and refined by respondent feedback and statistical analysis. Groups of questions addressing similar aspects of the concept are termed domains. Exploring the same concept through different domains increases reliability.

A questionnaire's ability to produce meaningful information is restricted to the population from which it was derived. Serious issues of transferability arise when there are changes in administration, language or culture.

Measurement scales

Quantitative responses are measured using the principles of psychometrics (the quantification of behaviour). The commonest scales are:

1. Visual analogue. A vertical or horizontal line 10 cm in length on which the respondent places a mark corresponding to the degree of attribute or agreement.

2. Likert. Gradations from *strongly agree* to *strongly disagree.* Usually an odd number (so the central response is *neutral*) and 5 to 7 gradations; higher numbers do not improve precision.

Format

Each question must ask about one item only. The Likert format converts questions into attitude statements, phrased so that the respondent agrees or disagrees. Presentation includes unrealistically positive and negative statements to avoid 'ceiling' and 'floor' effects. A ceiling effect is an artificially imposed upper limit to the response. This might arise from *'The doctor tried to help me'*. Rephrasing as a 'maximalist' statement *'The doctor did everything humanly possible to help me'* raises the ceiling. A floor effect is an artificial lower limit, avoided by the 'minimalist' statement *'The doctor did absolutely nothing to help me'*.

Respondents are more likely to agree than disagree. They may provide an appeasing answer, answer neutral for all, or give random responses. These vagaries are minimized by clear instructions, interspersing positive and negative items, and reversed statements (which ask the same question twice, once as a positive statement and once as a negative statement).

Critical appraisal

Questionnaires should reference their methodology (including literature review). This can be appraised like any other paper. Studies should justify the selection of a particular questionnaire. Instruments are judged by their responsiveness, reliability, reproducibility and validity within the study population.

- **Responsiveness**, expressed as an effect size, reflects sensitivity to meaningful changes.
- **Reliability** describes how much confidence can be placed in the findings. Longer questionnaires and larger populations enhance reliability.
- **Reproducibility** (or stability) is a population- and time-sensitive measure of duplicating results.

Two statistical tools quantify reliability and reproducibility:

1. Pearson's correlation coefficient 'p' describes relationships between items, e.g. test–retest correlation, or the relationship between specific variables and outcome. Values lie between −1.0 (negative correlation) to +1.0 (positive correlation). The larger the number, the greater the correlation. Coefficients of at least 0.7 are expected for group comparisons and in excess of 0.90 for individual comparisons.

2. Cronbach's 'α' measures internal consistency within a questionnaire. Values are from 0 to 1. Larger numbers indicate greater consistency. Values below 0.70 imply questions are unrelated; values above 0.90 suggest questions are too similar.

Validity is a more qualitative property, assessed by the following criteria:

1. Face validity describes whether 'on the face of it' the instrument appears to be an appropriate tool for the intended purpose.

2. Content validity assesses how completely the questionnaire covers the intended subject matter.

3. Criterion validity judges the instrument's relationship to any existing 'gold-standard'.

4. Construct validity explores the questionnaire's ability to measure changes predicted by the *construct* (theory) being studied.

Sources of error

Robust data are only obtained when a questionnaire is validated and has psychometric evidence to support its use within a specific culture for a specific purpose. Populations that are unrepresentative, small, or have poor response rates compromise results. Recall bias is influenced by the specificity of questions and time scale between event and questionnaire. Other variables, such as satisfaction, can also influence responses. Investigator objectivity is essential when interpreting any qualitative answers.

Administration

Results are more positive from investigator-administered questionnaires. These are time consuming, but allow greater exploration of issues. Uniformity of administration and recording is important. Self-administration is efficient, but requires clear instructions. The anonymous format encourages frank responses, particularly for sensitive issues. Postal questionnaires have higher numbers of omitted questions and lower response rates. This method is convenient, but is inappropriate for some populations.

Respondent considerations

The target population should be involved in questionnaire design. Evidence of clarity (e.g. reading age), completion time, and respondent acceptability (rate of returned questionnaires and omitted questions) should be included. The instrument should not place an emotional or physical burden on respondents.

Example

Baker's *Consultation Satisfaction Questionnaire* (*British Journal of General Practice* 1990; **40:** 487–490) exemplifies the painstaking process of development. Domains of satisfaction (general, professional care, depth of relationship and perceived time) were identified through open questions (face validity). A library of 126 statements was then refined by factor analysis for discriminatory value over the course of six field trials (content validity). The resulting self-administered 18 questions take 2–3 minutes to answer after a consultation. They include maximalist, minimalist and reversed statements. The unanswered question rate is 1%.

Cronbach's α is 0.91 overall, and test–retest correlation is 0.82–0.93 across the domains. Subsequent trials confirmed construct validity and appropriateness for postal-administration (*Quality in Health Care* 1992; **1:** 104–108), patient acceptability (*British Journal of General Practice* 1995; **45:** 249–253), and criterion validity (*Family Practice* 1996; **13:** 41–51).

Although the instrument has been validated on 11 000 patients, the principal criticism is that the questionnaire was developed on a population in the southwest of England, which excluded major urban areas. The questionnaire is now dated. Both of these factors need to be considered when interpreting results.

Further reading

Fitzpatrick R, Davey C, Buxton MJ, Jones DR. Evaluating patient-based outcome measures for use in clinical trials. *Health Technology Assessment* 1998; **2** (14).

Wensing M, van de Vleuten C, Grol R, Felling A. The reliability of patients' judgements of care in general practice: how many questions and patients are needed? *Quality in Health Care*, 1997; **6:** 80–85.

Related topics of interest

Critical appraisal (p. 70); Health status measurement (p. 119); Sampling and applicability (p. 130).

SOURCES OF INFORMATION

Richard J. McManus

Searching the published literature for articles is a key aspect of evidence-based medicine. When considering an EBM question or topic it is important to think about which sources of information are likely to be the most appropriate. For very important questions, a thorough search of multiple sources is needed, but in many cases a 'quick and dirty' search will be all that is required. Three main sources of information exist: paper (largely journals or books); electronic databases and electronic versions of paper publications; and experts.

Topics with a well established literature, such as hypertension or upper respiratory tract infection, are well represented in electronic databases. For more specialist or novel topics then either hand searching or asking an expert (useful in fast changing fields) will be more important. Secondary publications such as Bandolier or Clinical Evidence summarize and comment on primary research findings. These secondary publications can provide quick answers to many questions but they may reflect bias of the reviewer.

Hand searching

Hand searching is the 'gold standard' of searching methods. It involves physically reviewing paper copies of books or journals to determine whether they contain an article of interest. This can be very time consuming as relevant topics may exist in many different sources. The Cochrane Collaboration has performed hand searches of specific journals for randomized controlled trials. These have been logged and can now be accessed via the Cochrane Library Database. Very few questions will warrant an individual hand search.

Asking experts

For some questions, particularly in specialized or fast-moving areas, asking an expert may be an effective strategy (*BMJ* 1998; **317**: 1562–1563). Experts will usually be aware of ongoing research and of unpublished studies, the so-called 'grey literature'. This is particularly important in emerging or new fields where databases may not have appropriate indexing terms. Experts may be biased therefore they should not be the sole source of information.

Experts may include colleagues, researchers or even patients who often know much more about their own illness than their doctors. If an expert cannot be identified then it may be possible to locate one through the National Research Register. This is an online database of ongoing research in the UK that includes details of lead investigators and their research. A few clicks may be all that is required to find 'someone who knows'.

Electronic databases

Electronic databases are the heart of any literature search as they allow hundreds of thousands of articles to be searched simultaneously in seconds. Many now have links to the original articles which can be read online during a search. Different databases cover different areas. The ubiquitous Medline is the database most suited to doctors and will be as far as most of us get. Searching electronic databases requires care as even experienced searchers may only find about half of the relevant articles present on a given database. Librarians are information specialists who have the expertise to help refine a search. The difference they make can be quite surprising.

Many different databases are available. The choice depends on the subject matter and access. The following is a list of common databases.

1. Medline. The pre-eminent general medical database produced by the National Library of Medicine can be accessed via a number of different 'front ends' including PubMed, Ovid and Silver Platter. It includes more than 10 million citations from 4000 medical journals, about two-thirds with abstracts. The database starts from 1966 and is continuously updated with records sent direct as soon as they appear in print. Some journals, including the *BMJ*, can be accessed directly from citations within the PubMed version of Medline.

2. Embase. Embase consists of three linked databases: The main Excerpta Medica Database (another general biomedical database) and two more specialized subsets covering drugs, pharmacology and psychiatry.

3. CINAHL. The Cumulative Index to Nursing & Allied Health (CINAHL) database specializes in literature relating to nursing and allied health professions. Most articles are in English.

4. psychLIT. PsychLIT is a database produced by the American Psychological Association that covers psychological journals and books from 1887 to the present. It contains medical and psychiatric citations that include foreign language articles.

5. Web of science. This contains four relevant databases. A major advantage of these databases is the ability to do citation searches. This involves looking for articles which have cited a study that you are interested in. This is the reverse process of looking at the reference list of a study for related articles. It may discover articles not identified with traditional searching methods. The science citation index covers 5700 scientific journals (17 million articles) from 1973. The social sciences citation index is particularly good for qualitative research and it has 1725 indexed journals spanning 50 disciplines. Articles are available since 1981. The BioSciences and Clinical Medicine indexes contain further relevant articles from 1989 onwards.

6. ERIC. The ERIC database contains over 850000 citations to articles about education. It also contains some unpublished educational material.

7. Cochrane Library. The Cochrane Library consists of a collection of databases including: Database of Systematic Reviews; Database of Abstracts of Reviews of Effectiveness; The Cochrane Controlled Trials Register; and the Cochrane Methodology Register. See the Cochrane Collaboration chapter for further information.

8. Conference abstracts. Many conference abstracts, particularly from the USA are available on CD ROM. The index to scientific and technical proceedings indexes many large international conferences and conventions in a wide range of scientific disciplines and is available through the Web of Science (see above). It contains details of author, title and abstract, and where the abstract was presented.

9.   Eprint servers.   A recent addition to the electronic forum is the concept of electronic repositories for new research. In an idea borrowed from physics, researchers are being encouraged to post new research on the internet to allow online peer review before publication in print. Some journals are resisting this and consider it prepublication. However, it seems likely that in the future there will be a large database of all published work which will be subdivided by speciality and journal type (e.g. ejournal *vs.* conventional journal). The ejournals are likely to add value by acting as quality filters and a platform for commentaries and exchange of views.

10.   SIGLE.   System for information on Grey Literature in Europe (SIGLE) contains 'grey' literature from a wide variety of sources (conferences etc.) that is otherwise unavailable.

11.   Guidelines.   Guidelines are available on a wide range of topics. The best are evidence-based and examples of these include the North of England Guidelines Group (often published in the BMJ) and its Scottish Equivalent SIGN (Scottish Intercollegiate Guidelines Network – see below for link). Good guidelines will rate evidence quality for each recommendation (systematic review to consensus statement). Inevitably some guidance will have no evidence base and will rely on consensus between a group of experts as to 'best practice'. Where this has occurred, authors should be explicit. Guidelines should be clearly marked with the date of production and anticipated revision date. Guidelines can be searched for in Medline using the MeSH term 'Guidelines'.

12.   Others.   Other databases include Allied and Alternative Medicine, AIDSLINE and Toxline. Some search engines such as Medical Smart Search will search multiple databases at once (in this case Cochrane DARE database, Medline, the Merck manual and a guideline database). If in doubt, ask your librarian.

Further reading

Chalmers I, Altman DG. *Systematic reviews.* BMJ Publications, London, 1995.
Dawes M, *et al. Evidence-based practice: a primer for health care professionals.* Churchill Livingstone, Edinburgh, 1999.

Related topics of interest

Sources of information (p. 57); Sites of interest on the World Wide Web (p. 60); The Cochrane Collaboration (p. 67); The future of EBM (p. 150).

SITES OF INTEREST ON THE WORLD WIDE WEB

Richard J. McManus

The internet, or world wide web, is a rich source of medical information. However, as with anything on the internet, care must be exercised interpreting this information because it has not usually been subject to a rigorous evaluation process. Nevertheless, there are some very informative sites, many of which have been set up by well informed patient groups (e.g. **http://www.haemophilia.org/**).

Many journals publish electronic versions which can be accessed via the web. These often allow searching within a particular journal or across a number of related journals. The following is a list of useful sites. It is by no means comprehensive and some sites may change or disappear completely.

E-journals

Many journals are now available electronically. Table 1 summarizes links to some key, general journals.

Table 1

Journal	Web address	Notes
BJGP	http://www.rcgp.org.uk/	Mainly abstracts but some full text.
BMJ	http://www.bmj.com	Free access, searchable, full text with PDF.
JAMA	http://www.ama-assn.org/public/journals/jama/jamahome.html/	Free abstracts and some full text to non subscribers.
Lancet	http://www.thelancet.com/	Free abstracts and some full text for non subscribers.
NEJM	http://www.nejm.org/	Free abstracts and some full text to non subscribers.
PubMed Central	http://www.pubmedcentral.nih.gov/	PubMed Central is a web-based archive of a growing number of full text articles provided by publishers and directly linked to Medline.

Online databases

*1. **Medline.*** PubMed provides free access to Medline including publisher supplied citations which appear as soon as the article is in print. Web address: **http://www.ncbi.nlm.nih.gov/entrez/query.fcgi**

Medline Plus: This is available free to all BMA members at: **http://ovid.bma.org.uk/**

2. Embase. This can be accessed free of charge by BMA members at http://ovid.bma.org.uk/

3. Web of science. Subscription is required for access to science citation index, social sciences citation index etc. **http://wos.mimas.ac.uk/**

4. National research register. The online database of all UK research. http://www.doh.gov.uk/research/nrr.htm

5. UK library search. Online catalogue of UK university libraries: http://copac.ac.uk/copac/

Other online EBM resources

1. ARIF (Aggressive Research Intelligence Facility). ARIF is a team based in the West Midlands that searches out evidence in response to requests from local and regional providers. Their reports are available at: **http://www.hsrc.org.uk/links/arif/arifhome.htm**

2. Bandolier. Bandolier is a monthly compendium of a wide variety of EBM topics from methodology to the latest reviews. It is an excellent source of readable material written by people with a sense of humour **http://www.jr2.ox.ac.uk/Bandolier/**

3. Cochrane Collaboration. **http://hiru.mcmaster.ca/COCHRANE/default.htm** Web sites for individual Cochrane groups can be found at: **http://www.cochrane.org/cochrane/ccweb.htm#CRG**

4. Clinical Evidence. Clinical Evidence is a relatively new publication consisting of evidence on the effectiveness of clinical interventions. It is available in print (six monthly) and via the web: **http://www.clinicalevidence.org**. For mainstream topics it is quickly becoming indispensable. It should eventually become more comprehensive, if unwieldy!

5. Doctors.net. Most doctors will have had a flier from doctors.net through the door but the site is worth a visit as it provides free access to Cochrane and Medline. While you're there you can look up old colleagues . . . **http://www.doctors.net.uk/**

6. Evidence Based Medicine. This consists of summaries of important biomedical articles together with structured critiques and is a joint publication between the BMA and ACP journal club. It is available on CD ROM as Best Evidence and provides some articles free at the following site: **http://www.acponline.org/journals/ebm/ebmmenu.htm**

7. HTA. The Health Technology Assessment Programme supports high quality primary and secondary research and publishes full text reports on everything it commissions. These, and a number of systematic reviews, can be found at **http://www.hta.nhsweb.nhs.uk/**

8. Journals scan. Journal scan contains articles from journals and web sites that provide evidence for treatment, diagnosis or prognosis of medical conditions. These are presented in a question and answer format. **http://www.uaeu.ac.ae/jscan/**

9. National Electronic Library (NELH). This site is still in its infancy and is best viewed from within the NHSNet. It provides a wealth of evidence based information including access to Cochrane, Clinical Evidence and much more. **http://www.nhs.uk/nelh** One of the first sub branches of the NELH is the mental health section which can be found at: **http://www.nelmh.org/**

10. New Zealand Evidence Based Healthcare Bulletin. This bulletin summarizes news and information about evidence-based healthcare activities in New Zealand. **http://www.nzgg.org.nz/news/bulletin.cfm**

11. NHS Centre for Reviews and dissemination (NHS CRD). The publishers of effectiveness matters (regular updates on the effectiveness of important health interventions) and much more. **http://www.york.ac.uk/inst/crd/welcome.htm**

12. NHS Economic Evaluation Database. This site contains structured abstracts of economic evaluations. It is also produced by the NHS CRD. **http://agatha.york.ac.uk/nhsdhp.htm**

13. ScHARR Netting the Evidence Page. This contains a wealth of evidence-based material including further information on databases, search tools and useful software. It is an excellent link to other EBM sources. **http://www.nettingthe-evidence.org.uk**

14. Scottish Clinical Information Management in Primary Care. This site provides access to the 'SIGN' and other evidence-based clinical guidelines. **http://www.whow.scot.nhs.uk/scimp/**

15. Translation sites. Sites such as **www.babelfish.com/translations.shtml** allow instant translation via the web and can be useful in getting the gist of foreign language articles. These translations are not perfect but, if accompanied by some basic knowledge, are a lot quicker and cheaper than formal translation.

16. Other useful links. Any list of www links will never be comprehensive and may quickly become out of date. For a more extensive list than space allows, try the Bandolier links list at: **http://www.jr2.ox.ac.uk/Bandolier/bandlink.html**

Related topics of interest

Sources of information (p. 57); The Cochrane Collaboration (p. 67).

SEARCH STRATEGIES FOR ELECTRONIC DATABASES

Richard J. McManus

The results of any EBM search depend on the strategy used. Some strategies may seem daunting at first, but they can all be broken down into simple parts. In order to understand how searching an electronic database works, it is worthwhile reviewing how databases are organized.

Database organization

Electronic databases are arranged so that each aspect of an article's citation (title, authors, year, journal, when it first appeared in the database, abstract etc.) forms a separate field or sub field within the database. Each field can be searched individually for a specific item (e.g. author's name) or for a combination of items. For example, author X, in year Y, in journal Z. In addition, the fields can be searched for individual text words.

MeSH headings

Medical Sub Headings or MeSH terms are used by Medline and other databases as an additional form of indexing. MeSH headings allow articles sharing a common subject to be grouped together. This searching technique minimizes the chance of missing an article on a particular topic which does not happen to mention that topic in the title or abstract. MeSH headings have the disadvantage that they depend on the author or indexer choosing appropriate terms.

MeSH headings are arranged in a hierarchical structure. For example angina pectoris is a subdivision of coronary disease that is itself further subdivided into variant angina, unstable angina and syndrome X.

Each MeSH heading can be further subdivided into a number of different sub-headings which appear as suffixes – e.g. therapy or diagnosis. The use of MeSH headings within a search varies between database systems. Some (such as PubMed) use MeSH headings automatically whereas others (e.g. OVID) require choices to be made. If automatic MeSH searches are being used then it is worth checking (e.g. using 'details' in PubMed) exactly what terms are being used.

Simple searching

At the simplest level a search can be performed looking for individual terms, one at a time. This is, however, time consuming and can lead to unwieldy results containing thousands of 'hits'. A more efficient method is to combine individual terms with three different operators: AND, OR and NOT.

- AND: includes only articles appearing in both terms.
- OR: includes articles appearing in either term.
- NOT: includes articles appearing in one term but not the other.

These can help to focus a search down to relevant articles. Care must be taken because it is easy to unwittingly exclude useful studies particularly when using NOT.

Limiting search results

Searching often results in a large number of apparently relevant citations. In this case a method of focusing down is required to limit the results. Some databases have a specific feature to allow you to do this (e.g. *Medline*), others will require manual limiting. In either case there are a number of ways of limiting search results:

1. *Limit by date.* You may only be interested in relatively recent articles, particularly in a field such as near patient testing, where technological changes will quickly render studies obsolete. Similarly, if re-running a search, you may only be interested in articles appearing since the date of your last search.

2. *Limit by publication type.* A good meta-analysis is often ideal to answer an EBM question and can be specified as the publication type of interest. Similarly RCTs or articles with abstracts can be chosen.

3. *Limit by language.* Limiting by English language is commonly done but runs the risk of missing evidence not published in English. This may be appropriate for a 'quick and dirty' search but not for a systematic review.

4. *Limit by study population.* Age, gender and human/animal are all ways of further limiting results.

Increasing search results

Sometimes a search will be met with few or no relevant results. The strategy needs to be amplified in these cases:

1. *Exploding results.* Exploding a MeSH term does not refer to the damage frustrated searchers may inflict on their errant computers but rather a method by which all terms below a given term in the MeSH hierarchy are searched as well as the individual term. This is sometimes done automatically, but if not then it can quickly increase the number of hits from a search.

2. *Synonyms.* Use different terms for the same thing and combine using the OR operator – for example Thrush OR candidiasis OR monilia.

3. *Wild cards.* These are characters such as *, # or ? which allow either individual letters or whole sections of words to be varied. This is particularly useful in the case of American spellings (e.g. colour *vs.* color) or for some plural forms (e.g. women *vs.* woman). Separate wild cards apply for unlimited or limited numbers of characters, and mandatory or optional characters. Wild cards vary from system to system (PubMed, OVID etc.) so check the 'Help' if you want to use them. *Example* (Using OVID wild cards): woman.mp (key word search) gives 58 197 hits whereas wom?n.mp increases this to 271 022.

4. *Related articles.* This is a feature of a growing number of databases where an automatic system will look for similar articles to the one of interest. It has the advantage of speed but the disadvantage of being a little difficult to understand exactly what is being looked for.

Citation searching

The web of science databases (amongst others) allows citation searches. These can be very useful for tracking down articles because they allow automatic searching of secondary citations (those cited by a particular work).

Advanced searching

In some instances only a particular kind of study will be of interest. Various search 'filters' can be used automatically or, in some cases, be typed in. Cochrane speciality groups have devised strategies to find particular types of articles which are available from their website (see below).

The PubMed Version of Medline enables specific searches for articles about therapy, diagnosis, aetiology and prognosis using the 'clinical queries' tool. The strategies are based on the work of Brian Haynes (*Journal of the American Medical Informatics Association* 1994; **1**(6): 447–458) and can be optimized for either sensitivity or specificity.

Examples

The first two of these examples were done using Medline and the third using the Science Citation Index.

1. Searching with a single term. As explained above, this can often result in huge numbers of studies. For example, 'oral contraceptive' results in over 100 000 hits. One of the few instances where one term is often sufficient is a search for an individual. Try putting the name and initials of a colleague who has published some research and see what happens.

2. Combining terms. A patient tells you of a newspaper article that suggests taking simvastatin will reduce their risk of dementia. Dementia alone gives over 53 000 hits and statins 745. Combining statins AND dementia results in two articles, one from the *Lancet* and the other, a news article in the *BMJ* referring to the *Lancet* article. The *Lancet* article refers to a case–control study done using a general practice morbidity and prescribing database. It gives a relative risk for dementia in those taking a statin of 0.29 (95% CI 0.13–0.63) (*Lancet* 2000; **356:** 1627–1631).

3. Citation searching. You decide to look for papers about the validity of routinely collected health data (you want to know how accurate the figures in the dementia study are) and get nowhere with Medline because of problems with indexing. A colleague reminds you of a key *BMJ* article about the General Practice Research Database (GPRD – formerly VAMP) (*BMJ* 1991; **302:** 766–768). A search for the study on the Science Citation Index allows you to access the 161 papers that have cited it since 1991. This is a neat way of overcoming indexing problems.

Further reading

Greenhalgh T. *How to read a paper: the basics of evidence based medicine.* London: BMJ publications, 1997.

Sackett DL, Richardson WS, Rosenberg WMC, Haynes RB. *Evidence-based medicine: how to practice and teach EBM.* London: Churchill Livingstone, 1996.

Related topics of interest

Sources of information (p. 57); The Cochrane Collaboration (p. 67).

THE COCHRANE COLLABORATION

William S.M. Summerskill

The Cochrane Collaboration epitomizes evidence-based medicine. Archie Cochrane's compassion and practice of patient-centred medicine is promoted by providing systematic reviews of clinical effectiveness to enhance patient care. The collaboration is characterized by international cooperation and a multi-disciplinary approach involving all stakeholders including consumers. Systematic reviews use standardized, transparent methods with explicit review criteria in order to minimize bias. They are peer-reviewed and updated regularly.

Organization

The first Cochrane centre opened in Oxford in 1992. There are now dozens of centres involving hundreds of collaborators around the world. Collaborators are organized into specialist review groups based on clinical interests and skills. The Cochrane Consumer Network provides an interface for distributing findings to health care users. The Cochrane library publishes four issues per year, which are available by CD-ROM or Internet access. The library includes the following resources:

1. The Cochrane database of systematic reviews is designed to be a 'one-stop' source of dependable evidence. The reviews address significant clinical questions and consider all types of methodology, whether or not the study has been published. Explicit criteria (for searches, inclusion and analysis) are applied to the trials, from which evidence is considered for clinical recommendations. Each review includes an extensive bibliography of related research. Reviews in progress are listed as protocols. They describe clinical questions under study, list the reviewers, methodology, references and contact details, along with an expected date of publication.

2. The controlled trials register (CCTR) was established to provide a reliable index of trials, since half of all RCTs are not retrievable by advanced *Medline* searches. The register has been developed in conjunction with *Medline* and *Embase*, but also includes studies not listed in these databases. The purpose of the CCTR is to facilitate access to previous investigations. This helps to direct future research and minimize duplication.

3. Database of abstracts of reviews of effectiveness (DARE) provides a register of effectiveness reviews compiled by external sources. The abstracts give publication details and a structured presentation of methodology and findings.

4. Cochrane methodology register contains articles about different types of methods and analyses.

5. NHS economic evaluation database is a compilation of cost-effectiveness studies. This site can be accessed independently via the *NHS Centre for Reviews and Dissemination* (http://agatha.york.ac.uk/nhsdhp.htm).

6. Health technology assessment database assesses various interventions from economic, social and ethical perspectives to ensure quality and cost-effectiveness.

Searches

Databases can be searched by keyword with or without Boolean operators. A menu of 'hits' indicates the number of matches by category of article (systematic review, controlled trial register, DARE, etc.). Alternatively, abstracts can be browsed by category. Relevant reviews can be downloaded, printed, or ordered from the Cochrane centre in San Diego. The quarterly *Cochrane Library Journal* joined the *Medline* Database in 2000 and can be searched as a journal title.

Example

Corticosteroids given to mothers in premature labour reduce the risk of respiratory distress syndrome by 50% (OR 0.49; 95% CI: 0.41–0.60) and neonatal death due to prematurity by 40% (OR 0.59; 95% CI: 0.47–0.75). The first RCT evidence supporting this intervention was published in 1972, yet like dozens of other examples in medicine, patients continued to suffer (and die) unnecessarily, because the research information was not implemented in practice. It was almost 20 years later that this 'old-fashioned' intervention was implemented routinely for premature labour (*British Journal of Obstetrics and Gynaecology* 1990; **97:** 11–25). The Cochrane logo depicts a meta-analysis forest plot of the first seven RCTs comparing maternal corticosteroids and placebo to reduce mortality from prematurity (Figure 1). Whereas five of the seven trials included the vertical 'no benefit' line, the pooled data (represented by a diamond) confirms a significant benefit.

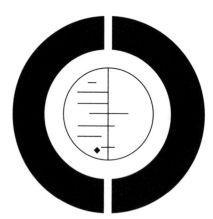

Figure 1. Cochrane Collaboration logo. (See text for details; reproduced with permission from the Cochrane Collaboration.)

Application

Systematic reviews from the Cochrane Collaboration are synonymous with evidence. They are authoritative and can be accessed rapidly. Cochrane reviews can form an integral part of grant applications, defence of service provision or a basis for changing clinician or patient behaviour. A patient handout based on a Cochrane systematic review of antibiotic prescribing for otitis media resulted in reduced prescription rates in a suburban London general practice (*BMJ* 1999; **318:** 715–716).

Interpretation

Evidence-based medicine encourages a critical appraisal of any source of data. It is important to maintain this approach even when considering a Cochrane review. Jadad *et al.* searched *Medline, CINAHL, Health Star, Embase* and the Cochrane library for systematic reviews and meta-analyses on the treatment of asthma (*BMJ* 2000; **320:** 537–540). When the 50 hits were reviewed, 40 had serious methodological errors. Of the 10 most rigorous reviews, seven were from the Cochrane library. Overall, Cochrane reviews achieved a higher quality score that those from peer-reviewed journals ($p < 0.005$).

Although the Cochrane library is likely to be the single best approximation of current evidence, Cochrane reviews do not cover all clinical scenarios. Questions of interest to Cochrane review groups are not necessarily those of relevance to clinicians. Furthermore, Cochrane reviews are not without controversy, such as the report that albumen infusion increases mortality in critically ill patients (*BMJ* 1998; **317:** 235–240).

Cochrane reviews would be expected to fulfil all the criteria for a systematic review. The inclusion/exclusion criteria should be compatible with the population for which one is seeking evidence. If the date of the review excludes more recent studies, other sources should be considered. The Cochrane library is an excellent starting point, but should be considered an adjunct to, rather than a replacement for, other databases.

Availability

The Cochrane library is distributed by Update Software (www.update-software.com/clibhome/clib.htm). The abstracts of systematic reviews are available free-of-charge via the Internet website, but access to the full reviews and the library costs from £132 ($235) for a single user per year (2001 prices). On-line access is available from some health regions in the UK, and elsewhere via medical libraries. The CD-ROM version is designed for Microsoft Windows® and requires a rapid processor and generous memory.

Further reading

Jadad AR, Haynes B. The Cochrane Collaboration – Advances and challenges in improving evidence-based decision making. *Medical Decision Making* 1998; **18:** 2–9.
www.cochrane.de

Related topics of interest

Systematic reviews (p. 17); Search strategies for electronic databases (p. 63).

CRITICAL APPRAISAL

William S.M. Summerskill

The process of critical analysis has its origin in Aristotle's *Poetics*. Three of Aristotle's criteria are as relevant to contemporary health research as they were to the 4th century BC theatre. They are truth, validity and probability.

1. Truth. Are the conclusions substantiated by the data?

2. Validity. Is the methodology sound and appropriate?

3. Probability. Is the statistical analysis significant, or in the case of qualitative studies, are the findings cohesive?

Critical appraisal, the process of assessing truth, validity and probability in a publication, lies at the heart of evidence-based medicine.

The purpose of reading research papers is to enhance one's view or practice of medicine. The rationale for change should come not from the author, topic or conclusion, but from the evidence itself. The purpose of critical analysis is not nihilism, but to confirm that the results are valid, clinically significant and applicable to one's own practice.

Approach

The author, institution and journal are the first features a reader notices. In order to reduce bias, purists will review articles blinded to this information and begin with the methods section. A careful study of the methodology will indicate whether the rest of the paper is worth reading as a source of evidence. The following headings are typically included in a methods section:

1. Literature review. Including databases, MeSH terms, hand-searches and attempts to retrieve unpublished material. Some qualitative studies will omit a literature review on the grounds of bias.

2. Population. Who is included/excluded and why? How were they recruited? Was the selection method appropriate for the intended population and study design?

3. Allocation. The timescale between allocation and entrance to the study should be brief. How was allocation performed, if it was not truly random, why not? Were subjects and investigators 'blinded' to the allocated intervention?

4. End-points. Unequivocal, clinically meaningful, readily measured.

5. Follow up. Is the timescale appropriate for the purposes of the study? What provisions are made for missing subjects and missing data?

6. Analysis. Quantitative research begins with a power calculation, to ensure that the study has adequate recruitment to provide significant results. If the statistical tests seem unfamiliar or inappropriate their use should be explained and referenced. Is analysis on an 'intention-to-treat' basis for RCTs? Is the potential impact of missing data considered with a sensitivity analysis?

Qualitative research includes a clear understanding of the researcher's involvement and perspective. Does the choice of method(s) match the population and study objectives? Are the findings validated by participants and triangulation? If interview data are involved, has a second reader confirmed the themes?

Whatever methodology is adopted, the study must reflect the principles of that approach, or of each constituent approach in a multi-method study. The following considerations provide a starting point.

Quantitative methodologies

Specific aspects in design and interpretation are considered in the chapters dedicated to each trial type. Common pitfalls are listed below.

1. Meta-analysis. Are all trials asking a similar question on similar populations in a similar fashion (homogeneity)? Is publication bias addressed?

2. Randomized controlled trials. Ensure that the intervention and control populations are similar in all respects except the intervention. Add up participants in tables to confirm that everyone is accounted for and included in an 'intention to treat' analysis.

3. Cohort studies. Greatest bias arises from loss to follow-up. Rule of '5 and 20'. Five per cent loss is unlikely to affect findings; 20% loss is a serious threat.

4. Case–control studies. Controls must match study population, not the general non-diseased population.

Qualitative methodologies

In qualitative papers, one is concerned that the methodology is congruent with the theoretical perspective of the study, and that the methodology is adhered to.

1. Phenomenology. Detailed descriptions of individual experiences, collected by intense analysis of a few conversations.

2. Grounded theory. A proposed theory based on common experiences, arising from many interviews.

3. Ethnography. Incorporates interviews, observation and external records to explain a culture.

4. Action research. A participatory study to produce a model of a process or change.

After reading the methods section, one should have a clear idea of how the study is organized and analyzed. Specialist procedures for data collection or processing should be referenced adequately to reinforce a clear picture of the research. Only if one appreciates the process of data management, can one be confident in the actual findings. If alarm bells ring at this stage, don't ignore them – try to increase your understanding of the study, and if still unsure, apply this scepticism to any conclusions which are not substantiated by the findings.

All types of studies should be checked for ethical approval and source of funding. At all times be aware of potential sources of bias.

Numerous 'checklists' are available to help with critical appraisal for different types of articles. Many can be downloaded from the ScHARR website 'netting the evidence' (www.nettingtheevidence.org.uk). Others can be browsed on-line, such as the open access Cochrane Handbook (www.cochrane.org/cochrane/hbook.htm). Checklists provide a useful starting point as they help to identify omitted details, and it is often the 'unmentioned' details that raise concerns about research quality.

The purpose of critical appraisal is not to find faults in research, or to become cynical about publications. These are easy and unprofitable traps to fall into. Critical appraisal is a tool to understand research findings and the ways in which they may or may not help one's individual patients. Sometimes critical appraisal does uncover fatal flaws, more often it sets findings in relief, highlighting areas of illumination and shadow, from which more informed choices can be made.

Further reading

Greenhalgh, T. *How to Read a Paper: The Basics of Evidence Based Medicine.* London, BMJ, 1997.
Popay J, Rogers A, Williams G. Rationale and standards for the systemic review of qualitative literature in health service research. *Qualitative Health Research* 1998; **8:** 341–345.

Related topics of interest

STATISTICAL METHODS (OVERVIEW)

Roland M. Valori

Evidence-based clinical decisions depend on correct statistical interpretation of the evidence, whether it comes from primary or secondary research. Busy clinicians cannot be expected to maintain an understanding of medical statistics sufficient to know whether a particular statistical test has been used correctly. However, a basic understanding of statistical methods will make it possible to interpret the results of a study much more reliably. This overview provides simple explanations to commonly used terms and methods. It is not intended to be exhaustive, but rather to be an overview that may persuade readers to consult some of the excellent texts on medical statistics.

Types of data

There are three basic types of data: categoric, ordinal and interval.

1. Categoric data identifies categories such as male/female or blue/green/brown/grey/other colour eyes. When categoric data has an obvious order to it, it is referred to as **ordinal** data.

2. Ordinal data can be objective such as 'heavy drinkers, moderate drinkers, light drinkers or abstainers' if the categories are based on objective criteria such as units of alcohol consumed/week. Alternatively ordinal data may consist of subjective outcomes as in health status measurement questionnaires: I feel my health is 'very good', 'good', 'average', 'poor', 'dreadful'. Tests of proportions or frequencies are used on this type of data.

3. Interval data can be divided into two groups: **discrete** and **continuous**. 'Discrete' data refers to data that can only have certain numerical values such as number of bed days. 'Continuous' data, as its name implies, does not have discrete steps. Examples of continuous data are weight and height. There are two key properties of continuous data: the mean and variance. Interval data are usually tested by comparison of means. This can only be done if the data follow a normal distribution (i.e. the data are reasonably symmetrically distributed about the mean). If it does not, then it can be transformed to a normal distribution, or be subjected to non-parametric methods of analysis.

Transformation of data

Hypothesis testing of continuous data can only be done when the data follow a normal distribution such as for blood pressure or height. Unfortunately much clinical data are not normally distributed. When the data are not normally distributed it is often possible to transform the data to form a normal distribution which can then be subjected to hypothesis testing in the normal way. The data are transformed by applying a mathematical formula to each data point such as multiplication or division. If there is a direct relationship of the raw data to the transformed data it is called linear transformation. If there is not a direct relationship (as with logarithmic or reciprocal transformations) it is called a non-linear transformation.

Hypothesis testing

The traditional method of determining whether one set of data are different from another is hypothesis testing. By convention the investigator will usually assume the null hypothesis, which predicts that the two sets of data are from the same population and therefore not different. The probability that the null hypothesis is correct is then determined. This probability is referred to as the P value. A P value of 0.10 tells us that there is a 0.10 probability or 10% chance that the null hypothesis (that there is no difference) is correct. An arbitrary cut-off of 0.05 or 5% has been chosen to indicate that the null hypothesis can be reasonably rejected. If the P value falls below this level the observed difference is regarded as a true difference or a statistically significant difference. Of course there is a 5% chance that this inference is incorrect. This potential error is called a type I or alpha error.

Statistical significance is not synonymous with clinical significance. Statistical significance means that the two sets of data are different. Sometimes a statistically significant difference may be clinically irrelevant.

Type II or beta errors

Very often the P value will exceed the 0.05 cut-off and it will be assumed that there is no difference between the groups. However, there is a chance that a genuine difference between the groups has been missed. It is possible to calculate the probability that acceptance of the null hypothesis is wrong, just as it is possible to calculate the probability that its rejection is wrong. A slightly more generous cut-off of 0.10 is regarded as being enough to be reasonably sure that a difference between the groups has not been missed. This potential error (0.10) is called a type II or beta error.

Estimation and confidence intervals

A more modern approach to expressing the result of a trial is to use the mean and the 95% confidence interval. In an experimental study the mean difference between groups is actually just an **estimate** of what the difference would be if an infinite number of similar experiments could be done. The 95% confidence interval around this estimate tells us that there is a 95% chance that the true difference lies somewhere within this interval. Put another way the confidence interval gives us a range of values within which we can be 95% certain the true difference lies.

Non-parametric methods

When the data do not fit a normal distribution and the data cannot be transformed, then non-parametric methods must be used. This technique uses a ranking method to compare two sets of data. The data are combined and ranked and each data point is given a value according to its rank (i.e. one for the highest value, two for the second highest, etc.). The sum of the ranks for the two data sets are then compared. The P values for the difference between the sum of the ranks is determined by using tables for different sample sizes.

Comparing proportions

Proportions can be compared and subjected to hypothesis testing in much the same way as means. A different test statistic is used (chi-squared) but it is interpreted in the same way. Similarly, an estimation of the difference between two proportions using the 95% confidence interval can be determined. Comparisons of proportions and frequencies is very common in medical research.

Correlation and regression

These techniques are used to assess the strength of association between two variables, to predict one variable when the other is known, and also to compare the amount of agreement between two variables (usually in the context of comparing two diagnostic tests).

Correlation tests the strength of association by measuring the degree of scatter around an underlying linear trend in a scatter diagram of the two variables. The coefficient of correlation r has a value between +1 and −1. Zero indicates no correlation and +/− 1 indicates perfect positive correlation or perfect negative correlation. It is possible to subject the correlation coefficient r to hypothesis testing and to construct confidence intervals around it.

Regression describes the relationship between two variables. A regression line is the line that minimizes the sum of the squares of the vertical distances to the line of each data point. This gives the term 'least squares regression'. With this line it is possible to predict one variable from the other using the equation $Y = a + bX$, where Y is the dependent variable, X the explanatory variable, b the slope of the line and a the point the line intersects the Y axis.

Multiple regression

There are two special regression techniques: multiple linear regression and logistic regression. Multiple linear regression, as its name implies, is a technique used to summarize the relationship of one response variable to two or more explanatory variables. For example blood pressure (the response variable) might be predicted by a number of other factors such as age, weight, smoking, family history (explanatory variables). With multiple regression the response variable must be normally distributed, therefore multiple regression techniques cannot be used for dichotomous outcomes such as disease/no disease. Logistic regression is used for this.

Logistic regression gets around the problem of the response variable not being normally distributed by transforming a measure of the response variable: the odds ratio. The odds ratio (probability of disease divided by the probability of not having the disease) is transformed by taking its log, hence the term logistic regression. Thus logistic regression enables us to predict the probability of something occurring (e.g. lung cancer) using several predictor or explanatory variables (e.g. smoking, age, sex etc.).

Appraisal

It is very difficult to make a judgement on whether the statistics used in a study are the most appropriate and then to determine whether they were applied correctly. To a very large extent we are dependent on the editors of journals to detect inappropriate statistical methods. Nevertheless, a basic understanding of the fundamentals of medical statistics will enable the reader to detect the more obvious errors and be suspicious in less clear-cut situations.

Further reading

Altman DG. *Practical statistics for medical research*. Chapman and Hall, London, 1991.

Bland M. An introduction to medical statistics. Oxford, Oxford University Press, 1988.

Gardner MJ, Altman DG. Confidence intervals rather than P values: estimation rather than hypothesis testing. *BMJ* 1986; **292:** 746–750.

Kirkwood BR. *Essentials of medical statistics*. Oxford, Blackwell Scientific 1988.

Related topics of interest

The P value (p. 77); Relative risk, relative risk reduction and odds ratio (p. 79); Risk reduction and the number needed to treat (NNT) (p. 83); Confidence intervals (p. 87); The power of studies (p. 108); Health economics (p. 122).

THE *P* VALUE

Marcel Levi

In the results of most research reports and scientific articles the *P* value seems to play a pivotal role. A *P* value less or greater than 0.05 conventionally indicates whether the findings are statistically 'significant' or 'not significant' respectively. As discussed later in this chapter, this pivotal role of the *P* value is based upon a misconception of the 'significance' of the statistical analysis of data.

Statistical significance and clinical relevance

In some publications a *P* value of $<0.00\ldots1$ is presented (almost in a macho fashion) as a statement emphasizing the high degree of significance of the study results. This level of *P* value certainly means that there is **statistical significance** but does not necessarily mean that the results are **clinically significant**.

Example

In patients with peripheral arterial disease pharmacological interventions are often prescribed to postpone the need for more interventional procedures. One such pharmacological intervention is pentoxifylline, which it is claimed, improves blood flow. The potential beneficial effect of this therapy, however, has been a matter of intense debate. In 1992 the results of a clinical trial that addressed this topic were published. In this trial 40 patients with peripheral arterial disease were randomized to either pentoxifylline or placebo. A difference in blood viscosity was shown between the two groups and more importantly, the maximal pain-free walking distance in the patients receiving pentoxifylline was significantly longer than in those patients receiving placebo ($P < 0.001$). Based on this finding, the authors concluded that pentoxifylline was clinically effective in patients with claudication. However, close examination of the data reveals that the absolute difference in maximal walking distance between the groups was only three and a half feet, which most doctors (and more importantly their patients) would consider to be not clinically significant.

This example demonstrates that statistically significant results do not automatically equate to results that are clinically relevant. Conversely, a study showing a 50% reduction in mortality in patients with upper gastro-intestinal bleeding may not be statistically significant in view of the relatively low incidence of in-hospital death in these patients and potentially due to a too small sample size. However, such an effect may be highly clinically relevant, since upper gastro-intestinal bleeding is a very common disorder.

Hypotheses and the *P* value

The *P* value can be used to test study hypotheses; testing hypotheses begins with the null-hypothesis, which states that two interventions are equally effective. Following completion of the study the groups' results are compared; if the results from the separate groups are different, the null hypothesis may be rejected. However, such a difference in experimental results may also have been caused by chance instead of indicating a true difference. The *P* value represents the risk that the observed difference is caused by chance alone. A *P* value of <0.05 reflects that the chance that the null hypothesis is falsely rejected (i.e. the chance that we think that two groups are different, while they actually are not) is <5%. However, a P value of >0.05 does not automatically mean that the two groups are not different. A P value of >0.05 simply indicates that it is not certain whether the groups are different or not. The 'significance' value of 0.05 should not be 'set in stone'; some results may be so clinically relevant, that an uncertainty of 10% may be acceptable and thus a P value of <0.1 is sufficient. Conversely, in some situations more caution is warranted, which may render the threshold of statistical significance to a P value of <0.025 or <0.01. Surprisingly, these 'variable' P values and their significance are hardly ever encountered or discussed in the literature.

Pitfalls of the *P* value

As has been mentioned earlier, the absence of a P value of <0.05 does not mean that there is no difference between the groups. For example, in the reports of clinical trials many authors mistakenly publish that patient characteristics in each group at the start of the trial were not different, as confirmed by a 'non-significant' P value of >0.05. Since there is no null hypothesis to be rejected in this situation (in fact, the assumption is that the groups are comparable), there is no role for a P value here. Moreover, although a large P value may indeed indicate that there is no difference between the groups, alternative explanations may be provided by a too small sample size, a low incidence of the test result or too much variability in the observed parameter.

The P value does not convey any information about the magnitude of differences between groups. Furthermore, the P value is equally influenced by the precision of the study results. Hence, a small (but consistent) difference may be highly statistically significant and a very large difference may lack statistical significance due to a variability of the test result. The P value can only be considered as an instrument to express the statistical certainty of a detected difference.

Alternatives to the use of the *P* value

Many researchers and biomedical journals prefer the use of 95% confidence intervals to the use of the P value. Confidence intervals are covered in detail elsewhere in this book. Briefly, a 95% confidence interval reflects the range of differentiation that may be encountered in 95% of the cases if the experiment were repeated endlessly. Although 95% confidence intervals are commonly used, 90% or even 99% confidence intervals may be more relevant in certain situations.

Further reading

Altman DG, Bland JM. Absence of evidence is not evidence of absence. *BMJ* 1995; **311:** 485.

Feinstein AR. P values and confidence intervals: two sides of the same unsatisfactory coin. *J Clin Epidemiol* 1998; **51:** 255–260.

Gradner MJ, Altman DG. Confidence intervals rather than P values: estimation rather than hypothesis testing. *BMJ* 1986; **292:** 746–750.

Related topics of interest

Statistical methods (overview) (p. 73); Confidence intervals (p. 87).

RELATIVE RISK, RELATIVE RISK REDUCTION AND ODDS RATIO

Marcel Levi

Risks

Risk represents chance; usually the chance of an unwanted event. There are several ways to express risk, such as the relative risk, the odds ratio, the relative risk reduction or the absolute risk reduction. In this chapter, each of these dimensions will be discussed.

Example

Imagine a population of 100 patients with diabetes. Fifteen of these 100 patients have developed renal failure. An age- and sex-matched control population (without diabetes) consists of 100 subjects and three of these patients have developed renal failure. The following 2×2 table can be constructed.

	Renal failure	No renal failure
Diabetes	15	85
No diabetes	3	97

Since 15% of patients with diabetes have developed renal failure, the risk of renal failure in this sample of patients with diabetes is 0.15. Viewed in isolation like this, this figure is not very informative. However, since there is an appropriate control population, it is possible to relate this risk to a background risk. In this control population the chance of developing renal failure is 3%, hence one can calculate a **relative risk** for diabetics developing renal failure, i.e. 0.15/0.03 = 5. In other words, a patient with diabetes has a 5-fold increased chance of having renal failure than a control subject. We can also do the converse calculation; in patients without diabetes, the risk of getting renal failure is 0.03/0.15 = 0.2 when compared with diabetic patients. Relative risk is identical to **relative risk ratio** or **risk ratio**, two other terms that are frequently encountered in the literature.

Another term describing a type of risk is the **relative risk reduction**. The relative risk reduction expresses the per cent reduction in events in non-exposed (no diabetes) compared to exposed (diabetes) by calculating (1 − relative risk) × 100% = (1 − 0.2) × 100% = 80%. Hence, having no diabetes reduces the risk of getting renal failure by 80%.

Similarly, the difference between diabetics and non-diabetics may be assessed by subtracting the risk of controls from the risk of diabetics and relate this to the risk in diabetics: (0.15 − 0.03)/0.15 = 0.12/0.15 = 0.80, which is called the **attributable risk** (of diabetes in developing renal failure). In other words: of all causes that may lead to renal failure in diabetics, the diabetes is the responsible factor in 80%.

There is, however, a further method of looking at the data. Fifteen of 18 patients that have developed renal failure have diabetes (0.83) and 85 of 182 patients that have not developed renal failure have diabetes (0.47). Hence, the relative risk of having diabetes in patients who develop renal failure is only 0.83/0.47 = 1.8. This example illustrates that when a relative risk has been calculated it is very important to identify what exactly has been used as the denominator. In some situations, this is relatively easy (diabetes will produce renal failure and not the other way around) and this should also not cause problems in prospective trials, however, in some retrospective case–control studies this problem may lead to problems in the interpretation of the data. A solution to this is to use statistical methods that are independent of the choice of denominator. Calculating the **odds ratio** represents such a method. Ignoring the underlying algebra, the odds ratio may simply be calculated as:

	Condition B1	Condition B2
Condition A1	a	b
Condition A2	c	d

$$\text{odds ratio} = \frac{a \times d}{b \times c}$$

In this example the odds ratio represents the chance that condition A1 is associated with condition B1. The odds ratio is a convenient method to calculate risk independent of the 'direction' of the risk factor. An odds ratio of 1.0 means that there is no association. Odds ratios are typically published with 95% confidence intervals, to indicate the expected range of the odds ratio in 95% of the occasions if the experiment would have been repeated indefinitely. If this range does not include 1, the association is probably present. Calculating the odds ratio of having renal failure in patients with diabetes (Table 1) the result is $(15 \times 97)/(3 \times 85) = 5.7$. The 95% confidence interval is 1.7–19.0.

Relative risk, absolute risk and individual risk

Working with relative risks in everyday clinical practical is an art. Relative risks provide an estimate of the chances of an individual to develop an illness, complication or response to therapy. However, one should remember that these chances have been calculated from observations on large groups of patients and the result of the group, as a whole may not automatically apply to the patient that is presently sitting in front of you.

Example

An 18-year-old woman comes to see you because one of her friends recently developed a venous thrombosis of the leg while using oral contraceptives. This woman has never had a thrombosis but she uses the oral contraceptive pill (OCP) too and she has read in the newspaper that using the OCP may enhance her risk of venous thrombosis. You wonder how large the risk associated with the use of oral contraceptives actually is? From recent publications it is concluded that the relative risk of developing venous thrombo-embolism in users of the OCP is 4 to 7, as compared with women not taking the OCP. When you tell this to the patient she is horrified and tells you that she wishes to stop taking the pill. However, when you explain that the absolute risk of getting venous thrombo-embolism at her age is extremely small and that 4 to 7 times extremely small is still extremely small she is somewhat more at ease. In fact, you can tell her that the absolute risk of getting venous thrombosis at her age while on the pill is only 1 in 10000. Much reassured, she decides to continue the OCP. However, three months later she returns with a swollen and painful right leg, which turns out to be a venous thrombosis. At this time she tells you (in no uncertain terms!) that she is not much interested in the other 9999 women who take the OCP and did not develop venous thrombosis.

This example illustrates the difficulty in explaining chances to patients:

- Firstly, relative risks are not very informative if they are not translated into absolute risks.
- Secondly, chances 'translate' badly to individual patients who do (100%) or do not (0%) develop a disease, respond to therapy, and so on. A (very) low relative or absolute risk does not completely exclude the occurrence of a disease or a complication, which when it occurs in an individual translates to an individual risk of 100%.

Chances, odds and risks may be helpful when estimating the likelihood that something is going to happen or for the development of general guidelines for the management of groups of patients with a comparable situation but may be hard to apply to or explain to individuals (who are only concerned with their own outcome). There is no easy way around this problem except through proper explanation of the meaning of chances and risks to patients and tailored individual counselling.

The various study types (observational studies, RCTs) are prone to varying degrees of bias and so some authorities have suggested that the results of relative risks, relative odds etc. produced from these studies should be viewed with the appropriate levels of caution:

- Case–control studies are most prone to bias and a relative odds of the order of 4 should begin to arouse interest in an association.
- Cohort studies are less prone to bias and the corresponding relative risk should be of the order of 3.
- In theory RCTs are 'bias free' and so a significant relative risk of greater than 1 should be taken seriously.

These are not hard and fast rules and some flexibility should be applied (for example if the study is investigating a serious outcome such as death then the figures should be interpreted accordingly and the threshold for concern warranting further investigation should be reduced) and it is worth remembering that the results are not statistically significant (conventionally) if the 95% confidence intervals include 1.

Further reading

Feinstein AR. *Clinical epidemiology: The architecture of clinical research.* WB Saunders Company, Philadelphia, 1985.

Green L. Using evidence-based medicine in clinical practice. *Primary Care; Clinics in Office Practice* 1998; **25:** 391–400.

Hennekens CH, *et al. Epidemiology in medicine.* 1st Edition, Little Brown and company, Boston, 1987.

Related topics of interest

Risk reduction and the number needed to treat (NNT) (p. 83); Confidence intervals (p. 87); Explaining risks to patients (p. 145).

RISK REDUCTION AND THE NUMBER NEEDED TO TREAT (NNT)

Dermot P.B. McGovern

"Lies, damned lies and statistics"   *Mark Twain*

There are a number of valid statistical entities for the reporting of results from trials comparing different interventions. A recent addition to these is the concept of the number needed to treat (NNT) to prevent one adverse outcome and the number needed to harm (NNH). More traditional approaches convey data as the relative risk reduction (RRR) and the absolute risk reduction (ARR). The authors of interventional (comparative) studies may present the data as any one of these statistical modalities (but preferably as all three) and the modality they choose could have a significant effect on how the data are perceived.

To calculate the various modalities the controlled event rate (CER), which is the incidence of the study end-point in the control or placebo group and the experimental event rate (EER), the incidence of study end-point in the experimental (interventional) group, are necessary:

- The RRR can be calculated as the CER minus the EER all divided by the CER.

$$\frac{CER - EER}{CER}$$

- The ARR is simply the CER minus the EER.   (CER – EER)
- The NNT is the inverse of the ARR.   (1/ARR)

Imagine three different conditions that have a mortality of 70%, 7% and 0.7%, respectively and an intervention that reduces these to 35%, 3.5% and 0.35%, respectively. Table 1 demonstrates the relationship between the RRR, ARR and NNT in these circumstances.

Table 1. The relationship between the RRR, ARR and NNT calculated from different control event and experimental event rates

	CER	EER	RRR $\frac{CER - EER}{CER}$	ARR (CER – EER)	NNT (1/ARR)
Treatment 1	70%	35%	50%	35%	~ 3
Treatment 2	7%	3.5%	50%	3.5%	~ 29
Treatment 3	0.7%	0.35%	50%	0.35%	~ 286

Table 1 clearly demonstrates that the **relative risk reduction** does not discriminate between large and small absolute differences. In epidemiological terms treatment 1 would be far more important than treatment 3 (assuming similar disease prevalences) but the RRR does not indicate this. It is also clear that the RRR is similar for all 3 conditions despite the huge differences in the NNTs.

Trial results are commonly reported as the RRR as this makes them appear more impressive: e.g. the results from a single interventional trial were sent to healthcare purchasers expressed as a RRR, an ARR and a NNT. The purchasers were asked to rank the interventions in order of effectiveness. The majority ranked 'the one' expressed as the RRR as the most effective and only one replied (correctly) that in fact they were all identically effective. It will come as no surprise that pharmaceutical representatives/literature commonly present their drug's results as a RRR (and confusingly the RRR is often referred to as 'The Risk Reduction').

Despite these shortcomings the RRR does have a role especially when discussing therapy options with an individual patient. In the theoretical examples from Table 1 a patient could truthfully be told that compliance with treatment would reduce their chances of dying by 50% (for all three conditions).

The **absolute risk reduction** overcomes the problems associated with the relative values but is a very difficult value to 'visualize' and deal with. What does an ARR of 5% actually mean? The **number needed to treat** is essentially the same result as the ARR, but expressed in a more user-friendly manner. The NNT represents the number of patients who need to receive the intervention (compared to placebo/study comparator) to prevent one adverse outcome. One painful consequence of expressing the results as an NNT instead of an ARR is that it becomes all too obvious to doctors how ineffectual (in absolute terms) many interventions are.

Similar principles can be used to calculate the **numbers needed to harm** (NNH). This figure gives an idea of the adverse events associated with a treatment and is the inverse of the absolute risk increase (ARI). Together the NNT and the NNH can be combined to produce statements giving an idea of how effective, but at what cost, a treatment may be (see Example 1 for a worked example).

NNTs (and NNHs) can also be calculated from the results of meta-analyses either from calculating the ARR from the raw data or using a formula to calculate the NNT directly from the odds ratio (see Example 2 below for a worked example of this). It is very appropriate to calculate the NNT from meta-analyses as the results are usually expressed as odds ratios or relative risks, both of which are relative values and have similar weaknesses to the RRR.

A form of NNT, the numbers needed to screen (NNS) is increasingly appearing in the results of trials assessing the efficacy of screening. The NNS is calculated by a similar method as the NNT and represents the number of people who need to be entered into a screening programme in order for one of them to avoid the adverse outcome (usually death from the condition under question).

When quoting NNTs, it is important to remember to include information about the duration of time that the patient was exposed to the intervention in order to achieve the stated benefit. It is also relevant to include information about the length of follow up at which the risk reduction and NNTs were calculated.

All numerical values (including NNTs) obtained through clinical trials should be quoted with their confidence intervals (CI) (conventionally 95% CI) (see chapter on Confidence intervals).

A list of examples of NNTs for common interventions can be found in Table 2.

Example 1 (Low-dose aspirin and vitamin E in people at cardiovascular risk. *Lancet* 2001; 357: 89–95)

This study compared the efficacy, in a general practice setting, of low-dose aspirin against no-aspirin (placebo would have been better!) in the primary prevention of cardiovascular events in people with one or more major cardiovascular risk factors. The study also examined the efficacy of vitamin E but these (negative) results have been ignored for the purpose of this example. 4495 volunteers were randomized to receive no aspirin (control group) or 100 mg of aspirin (experimental group) and were followed up for a mean of 3.6 years. The results were

	CVS death	CVS event	Severe bleed
Aspirin (EER)	0.8%	6.3%	1.1%
No-aspirin (CER)	1.4%	8.2%	0.3%

For CVS events: $RRR = \dfrac{CER - EER}{CER} = \dfrac{8.2 - 6.3}{8.2} \sim 23.2\%$

$ARR = CER - EER = 8.2 - 6.3 = 1.9\%$

$NNT = 1/ARR = 1/0.019 \sim 53$

So 53 people with one or more major cardiovascular risk factors need to be treated with 100 mg aspirin for 3.6 years to prevent one cardiovascular event.

$$\text{For CVS deaths: } RRR = \frac{CER - EER}{CER} = \frac{1.4 - 0.8}{1.4} \sim 43\%$$

$$ARR = CER - EER = 1.4 - 0.8 = 0.6\%$$

$$NNT = 1/ARR = 1/0.006 \sim 167$$

So 167 people with one or more major cardiovascular risk factors need to be treated with 100 mg aspirin for 3.6 years to prevent one cardiovascular death.

It is also important to consider the adverse events that aspirin can cause (namely significant bleeding):

The absolute risk increase (ARI) = EER − CER = 1.1% − 0.3% = 0.8%.

The numbers needed to harm (NNH) = 1/ARI = 1/0.008 ~ 125.

So 125 people with one or more major cardiovascular risk factors need to be treated with 100 mg aspirin for 3.6 years to cause one significant bleed.

The NNT and NNH can be combined to produce an overall summary of the drug's effectiveness:

'If you treat a thousand people with one or more major cardiovascular risk factors with 100 mg of aspirin for 3.6 years you will prevent approximately six cardiovascular deaths (1000/167) and approximately 19 cardiovascular events (1000/53) at the cost of eight significant bleeds (1000/125)'.

Example 2

The use of tricyclic antidepressants (TCAs) to relieve pain in post herpetic neuralgia was examined in this systematic review (*Family Practice*, 1996; **13**: 84–91). The TCAs used were amitriptyline (two studies) and desipramine (one study). The pooled odds ratio for complete or large reduction in pain at the end of 3–6 weeks treatment was 0.15 (95% confidence intervals 0.08–0.27). This can be converted to an NNT using the following equation

$$NNT = \frac{1 - [PEER \times (1 - OR)]}{PEER \times (1 - OR) \times (1 - PEER)}$$

Where PEER is the Patient's Expected Event Rate (the rate at which the end-point (in this case pain relief) occurs in the control group) and OR is the odds ratio.

$$\text{The PEER in this meta-analysis} = \frac{\text{Number controls with pain reduction}}{\text{Total number of controls}} = \frac{7}{108} = 0.0648$$

$$\text{Hence the NNT} = \frac{1 - [0.0648 \times (1 - 0.15)]}{0.0648 \times (1 - 0.15) \times (1 - 0.0648)} = \frac{0.9449}{0.0515} = 18.3 \sim 18$$

Therefore, 18 patients with post herpetic neuralgia, need to be treated with tricyclic antidepressants for 3–6 weeks in order to produce complete or large reduction of pain in one of them.

Table 2. Examples of NNTs (a more comprehensive list can be found at the bandolier website – http://www.jr2.ox.ac.uk/Bandolier)

Intervention	Versus	Outcome	NNT
Simvastatin in coronary artery disease	Placebo	1 coronary death over 5 years	29
rtPA infusion in acute MI	Streptokinase	To save 1 life	100
30 days of 162 mg of aspirin daily following acute MI	Placebo	To save 1 life at 30 days	42
1.5 MU infusion of streptokinase after acute MI	Placebo	To save 1 life at 30 days	36
Streptokinase infusion & 30 days of aspirin after acute MI	Placebo	To save 1 life at 30 days	19
Enalapril in NYHA class IV congestive heart failure	Placebo	To prevent 1 death at 1 year	6
α interferon and ribavarin in chronic hepatitis C	α interferon alone	To clear virus at one year	4
Any antihypertensive for severe hypertension	Placebo	To prevent 1 stroke, MI or death in 1 year	15
Mammography & regular breast examination	No intervention	To prevent 1 death from breast cancer over 9 years	1075

Tables like this are often used to compare different interventions. This is not strictly correct as these values are mostly calculated from different studies performed on different populations, under different circumstances with different data retrieval methods.

Related topics of interest

Confidence intervals (p. 87); Meta-analysis (p. 19); RCT (p. 25).

CONFIDENCE INTERVALS

William S.M. Summerskill

Confidence intervals are estimates of where 'true' answers are most likely found. Whereas *p* values denote statistical significance, confidence intervals (CIs) indicate clinical significance. They aid the interpretation of research results in two ways: by describing the magnitude of a clinical effect and by providing limits to the (im)precision surrounding any value. CIs are customarily set at 95%, meaning that one can be 95% confident that the true value of a result lies within the given interval. The width of the interval reflects the precision (if narrow) or potential range (if broad) of the clinical effect.

Definition

The calculation of CIs depends on a representative sample from a normally distributed population. The width of the interval is determined by the degree of confidence desired (i.e. 90%, 95% or 99%), the variability of the data (standard error) and the number of observations (*n*). Larger numbers of observations result in narrower intervals. But for any number of observations, the greater the certainty desired that the true value lies within the interval, the broader that interval will be.

The simplest example of a confidence interval is for a mean. In a normal distribution, 95% of the values fall between −1.96 standard errors (SE) of the mean and +1.96SE. Figure 1 illustrates the confidence intervals surrounding the measurement of serum albumin in 100 random samples from patients with primary biliary cirrhosis

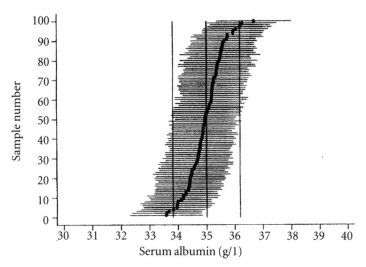

Figure 1. 95% CI for the mean albumin concentration in PBC, derived from 100 random samples. (Re-drawn from an original figure, in Altman DG. *Practical Statistics for Medical Research.* London: Chapman and Hall, 1997, reprinted with permission.)

(PBC). The mean value for serum albumin in this population is 35 g/l, with a 95% CI of 33.8–36.2 g/l. One would expect five of the 100 readings to fall outside the confidence interval (portrayed by vertical bars), and in fact four values are below this, the CI and three above. The CIs for these seven specimens do not include the mean of 35 g/l.

Application

The International Committee of Medical Journal editors have called for the use of confidence intervals to help explain the uncertainty of findings, because they convey more useful information than p values alone (*BMJ* 1988; **286:** 401–405). Confidence intervals can be calculated for correlation, costings, means, NNTs, ORs, risk, survival times, etc. – any value that is derived from continuous measurements on a normally distributed population.

Confidence intervals can also be used to estimate sample size when performing 'power' calculations. In the future, CIs may be applied to predict individual patient responses to different treatments (*Computers and Biomedical Research* 1998; **31:** 244–256).

Example

Various formulae are available for calculating CIs in specific situations. When different methods are used, slightly different estimates are obtained. To calculate the CI for NNT, one must consider the difference between two proportions (event rate in the intervention group and event rate in the control group), as illustrated in the example below. (Readers interested in obtaining CIs for NNTs painlessly can refer to the 'EBM toolbox' on the *Centre For Evidence-Based Medicine* website (http://cebm.jr2.ox.ac.uk/) where an on-line CI calculator is available.)

Does the prescription of antibiotics for sore throat medicalize a self-limiting condition (*BMJ* 1997; **315:** 350–352)? GPs in 11 practices tested this hypothesis by randomizing patients with sore throat and an abnormal physical examination to receive an immediate antibiotic, no antibiotic, or a delayed prescription for antibiotic to be collected if symptoms did not settle in three days. After 1 year, 69 out of 182 in the antibiotic-treated group (38%) re-presented with a new episode of sore throat, compared to 89 out of 328 of those not receiving an immediate antibiotic (27%).

How might these findings affect one's own practice? First calculate the ARR: $(P_2-P_1) = 0.38 - 0.27 = 0.11$ (or 11%). The 95% CI for the ARR is $11 \pm 1.96\text{SE}$. The SE is calculated from the proportional event rates ($P_1 = 0.27$, $P_2 = 0.38$) and the populations ($n_1 = 328$, $n_2 = 182$).

$$\text{SE} = \sqrt{\frac{P_1(1-P_1)}{n_1} + \frac{P_2(1-P_2)}{n_2}} = \sqrt{\frac{0.27(1-0.27)}{328} + \frac{0.38(1-0.38)}{182}} = 4.35\%$$

95% CI ARR $= 11 \pm (1.96 \times 4.35)$. ARR $= 11$ (95% CI: 2–19). As NNT is the reciprocal of ARR, the reciprocals of the ARR confidence interval provide the NNT CI. The ARR is $(0.38-0.27) = 0.11$, giving a NNT of $\frac{1}{ARR} = \frac{1}{0.11} = 9$. The 95% CI $= \frac{100}{19}$ to $\frac{100}{2}$ or 5 to 50. This is expressed as NNT $= 9$ (95% CI: 5–50). For ease of demonstration the numbers have been rounded off, a more accurate estimate is: NNT $= 9.3$ (95% CI: 5.2–44.6).

This means that one would have to withhold immediate antibiotics from nine patients with sore throat in order to prevent one patient from re-presenting at his/her next episode. One can be 95% confident that the actual number of patients will lie between 5 and 45. This nine-fold spread must be included when considering the implications of a policy change.

Interpretation

The usefulness of confidence intervals is their ability to set single values in perspective. A NNT of 6 with a 95% confidence interval of 2–8 is clearly more desirable than NNT = 6 (95% CI: 4–32).

If confidence intervals for continuous data overlap, this implies that there is no statistical difference between outcomes, since the null hypothesis is not disproved. However, CIs can help explain the results of trials or meta-analyses with p values greater than 0.05, as an estimation of possible 'true values' is presented. Because the width of a confidence interval reflects the sample size, a p value greater than 0.05 with a broad interval indicates that there *may* be a difference between populations, but that the study size was too small to demonstrate this (a type II error). A narrow CI in association with a p value >0.05 suggests that the findings are truly insignificant.

If a CI comparing ratios crosses one, then there is no statistically significant difference between outcomes, since the numerator and denominator are the same.

Confidence intervals can be misused, particularly if applied to small samples, when implausible values can be obtained. When groups are compared, the CI should describe the difference between groups, rather than the difference in intervals from each group.

Confidence intervals are only listed in a minority of papers at present, but their role in research is increasing. If contemporary studies do not incorporate confidence intervals, ask yourself 'why'? It may be because the numbers are small, or the results are widely scattered. If so, this insight has a bearing on interpreting the research findings.

Further reading

Altman DR, Machin D, Bryant TN, Gardner MJ. *Statistics with Confidence.* 2nd edn, Bristol, A. W. Arrowsmith Ltd, 2000.

Related topics of interest

SENSITIVITY AND SPECIFICITY

Marcel Levi

Sensitivity and specificity are terms that provide information about the accuracy of a diagnostic test. A diagnostic test is usually performed to establish the presence or absence of a disease. However, diagnostic tests are rarely 100% accurate and may give false-positive (i.e. the test indicates there is a disease, while this is in fact not true) or false-negative (i.e. the test falsely overlooks the presence of the disease) results.

Definitions

The **sensitivity** of a test reflects the proportion of patients with the disease that have a positive test result, out of the total number of patients with the disease. The **specificity** of a test reflects the proportion of healthy patients that have a negative test result, out of the total number of patients that do not have the disease.

Obviously, the sensitivity and specificity of a test can only be assessed when there is a means to definitively establish the presence or absence of the disease. The test in question then has to be compared with this '*gold-standard*' method in a sufficiently large consecutive sample of patients. Such a comparison allows for the construction of a 4×4 table in which a positive or negative test result can be compared with the actual presence or absence of the disease.

Example

Urine testing strips aim to rule out or in a urinary tract infection (UTI) without the need for a formal urine culture specimen being sent. The efficacy of one type of strip was tested in a Dutch study (*Family Practice*) 1995; **12**: 290–293). The strips in question measured blood, leucocyte activity and nitrite. For simplicity, this example will concentrate on the results for leucocyte activity on a dipstick compared with urine culture ($> 10^5$ organisms/ml), the "gold standard."

Sixteen GPs in 12 practices collected urine samples from 1388 patients with symptoms suggestive of a UTI. Each urine sample was tested with a dipstick prior to being sent for culture. In 77 cases, culture of these specimens was contaminated leaving 1311 cultures of which 906 (69%) were positive. Of these 1311 urine tests with a culture result, the dipstick gave 787 positive tests for blood. The results are tabulated below.

	MSU culture positive ($> 10^5$ bacteria/ml)	MSU culture negative	
Leucocyte activity present on dipstick	787	288	**(1075)**
No leucocyte activity present on dipstick	118	118	**(236)**
	(905)	**(406)**	**1311**

The sensitivity of the urine dipstick test is calculated by taking the proportion of patients with a positive urine culture that have leucocyte activity present on dipstick, i.e. 787/905 = 87%, which is fairly high. The specificity of the urine dipstick test can be calculated by taking the proportion of the patients without a positive urine culture that have a negative leucocyte activity dipstick test i.e. 118/406 = 29%, very low. In other words, in patients with urinary symptoms and UTI the leucocyte activity is usually positive (high sensitivity) but in many cases of urinary symptoms without UTI the test is also abnormal (low specificity).

Overall accuracy

The overall accuracy of a diagnostic test can be simply calculated by multiplying the sensitivity and the specificity. The overall accuracy of the D-dimer test for the diagnosis of venous thrombosis in the example is $0.97 \times 0.75 = 0.73$. This means that the test gives a reliable answer in 73% of the cases. Hence, the overall accuracy provides a global idea about the test performance but has limited value in estimating the exact place of a diagnostic test clinical practice, since some situations require 'exclusion' of a diagnosis and in some situations 'confirmation' of a diagnosis is more important. A test with a high sensitivity can be used to rule out diagnoses (i.e. if a test has 100% sensitivity and the test is negative then one can be sure that the patient does not have the disease), conversely if the test has a high specificity it can be used to rule in the diagnosis (i.e. if a test has 100% specificity and the test is positive then one can be sure that the patient does have the disease). Tests with high sensitivity and those with high specificity are useful in different situations; if it is important not to 'miss' a diagnosis then a test with a high sensitivity is optimal and if it is preferable not to get too many false positive results then a test with a high specificity is more useful.

Further reading

Jaeschke R, *et al.* Users guide to the medical literature. VI. How to use an article about a diagnostic test: B. What are the results and will they help me in caring for my patients. *JAMA* 1994; **271:** 703–707.
McGinn T, *et al.* Clinical prediction guides. *Evidence Based Medicine* 1998; **3:** 5–6.

Related topics of interest

Screening (p. 50); Negative and positive predictive values (p. 96).

LIKELIHOOD RATIOS

Marcel Levi

Likelihood ratios are helpful in determining how useful diagnostic tests will be. A likelihood ratio can predict how the result of a diagnostic test will transform the pre-test likelihood (i.e. the chance of having the disease, or in other words: the prevalence of the disease) to a post-test likelihood, i.e. the chance of having the disease knowing the test result. There are two likelihood ratios:

- The **positive likelihood ratio** is the likelihood ratio that should be applied when the test result is positive (or abnormal).
- The **negative likelihood ratio** is applicable when the test result is negative (or normal).

The positive likelihood ratio is the ratio obtained when the probability of a positive test in those who have the disease (the sensitivity of the test) is divided by the probability of a positive test in those who do not have the disease (which equals 1 – specificity). Similarly, the negative likelihood ratio is determined by the division of the chance of a negative test result in those with the disease (which is 1 – sensitivity) by the chance of a negative test result in those without the disease (which is the specificity). Hence:

$$\text{The positive likelihood} = \frac{\text{sensitivity}}{1 - \text{specificity}}$$

$$\text{The negative likelihood} = \frac{1 - \text{sensitivity}}{\text{specificity}}$$

The likelihood ratio can be used to calculate the post-test likelihood (in terms of post-test odds ratio) from the pre-test odds ratio using the following formula:

$$\text{Posterior odds} = \text{prior odds} \times \text{likelihood ratio}$$

However, use of this formula requires the translation of the pre-test likelihood (which is usually expressed as a percentage or a chance) to a pre-test odds and the calculation of posterior odds to post-test likelihood (in terms of chance or percentage). This is cumbersome and to facilitate the use of likelihood ratios, one can use a simple nomogram (Figure 1) that translates the pre-test likelihood into a post-test likelihood using likelihood ratios.

To use the nomogram, one should anchor a ruler at the given pre-test probability on the left axis and then pivot a ruler until it crosses the calculated likelihood ratio (either positive or negative). The post-test probability can then be read from the point where the ruler crosses the right axis.

Example

A 65-year-old man attends your surgery asking for a PSA test to screen him for prostatic carcinoma. He is asymptomatic and you think his chance of prostate cancer is 5% at most (these estimates can be based on epidemiological evidence but are often based on clinical judgement,

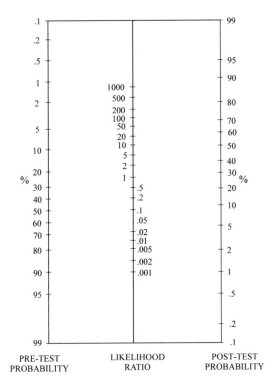

PRE-TEST PROBABILITY	LIKELIHOOD RATIO	POST-TEST PROBABILITY

Figure 1. Nomogram demonstrating the relationship between the pre-test probability, likelihood ratio and the post-test probability. (Reprinted from Sacket DL, *et al. Clinical Epidemiology: A basic science for clinical medicine*, 2nd edition, Little Brown and Company, Boston/Toronto, 1991, and adapted from Fagan TJ, Nomogram for Bayes' theorem. *N Engl J Med* 1975; **293**: 257).

i.e. how 'suspicious', on clinical grounds, are you that the patient has the condition?). You decide to find out how effective a PSA test is at detecting prostate cancer before agreeing to do the test. You do a quick Medline search and find a paper from Canada which reports a sensitivity and specificity of 80.7% and 89.6% respectively for a PSA > 3.0 mcg in asymptomatic men aged 45–80 years old (*Journal of Urology* 1992; **147**: 846–851). This fits with your patient so you assemble a 2 × 2 table as below

	Prostatic carcinoma	No prostatic carcinoma	
PSA ≥ 3.0 mcg/l	4	10	**(14)**
PSA < 3.0 mcg/l	1	85	**(86)**
	(5)	**(95)**	

The positive likelihood ratio of the PSA test for the diagnosis prostate cancer in asymptomatic men can be calculated by dividing the proportion of patients with a positive PSA who have the disease (4/5 = 0.8) by the proportion of patients with a positive PSA who do not have the disease (10/95 = 0.11) = 0.8/0.11 = 7.3. As you will see, this is identical (taking rounding errors into account) to the sensitivity (0.81) divided by 1–specificity (0.1). Using the nomogram with the estimated pre-test probability and calculated likelihood ratio one can calculate a post-test likelihood of a positive test result of about 25%. Hence, a positive test result will increase the probability of having prostatic carcinoma from 5% to 25%, which will certainly cause you to investigate this man more thoroughly (as shown in Figure 2).

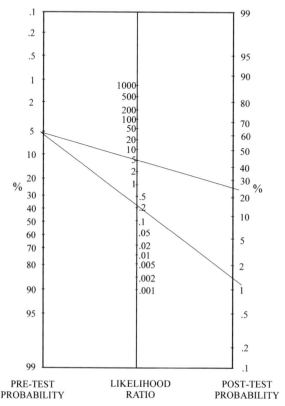

Figure 2. Nomogram for positive likelihood ratio for PSA in prostate carcinoma.

Similarly, the negative likelihood ratio may be calculated, as the ratio of the proportion of patients with a negative PSA who do have prostatic carcinoma ($1/5 = 0.2 = 1$–sensitivity) and the proportion of patients with negative PSA who do not have prostatic carcinoma ($85/95 = 0.90$ = specificity) = $0.2/0.9 \sim 0.22$. Using the nomogram, it is clear that a negative test result will render the post-test likelihood from 5% to 1–2%, which is less helpful.

Note that the likelihood ratio (like the sensitivity and specificity) is not influenced by the prevalence of the disease and may therefore be used in situations with different levels of pre-test likelihoods. Another major advantage of likelihood ratios is that they can be refined to various levels of test results. In this example we have used a 'positive' or a 'negative' PSA test around a cut-off point, but laboratories report PSA quantitatively rather than qualitatively and for each range of values a likelihood ratio can be calculated. In fact, a very high PSA titre is even more likely to be caused by the presence of prostatic carcinoma than a modestly elevated level. The use of likelihood ratios permits the refinement of several levels of the test result and may lead to a more precise estimate of the post-test likelihood of the presence or absence of the disease.

Further reading

Hagen EC, *et al.* Antineutrophil cytoplasmic antibodies: a review of the antigens involved, the assay, and the clinical and possible pathogenetic consequences. *Blood* 1993; **81:** 1996–2002.

Ingelfinger JA, *et al. Biostatistics in clinical medicine.* 3rd Edition. McGraw-Hill, Inc, New York, 1994.

Sacket DL, *et al. Clinical epidemiology: a basic science for clinical medicine.* 2nd Edition. Little, Brown, Boston, 1991.

Related topic of interest

Sensitivity and specificity (p. 90).

NEGATIVE AND POSITIVE PREDICTIVE VALUES

Marcel Levi

An alternative method to the sensitivity and the specificity of expressing the accuracy of a test is by calculating the *positive* and *negative predictive values* of an abnormal and a normal test result, respectively. The positive predictive value of a test indicates the proportion of patients with an abnormal test result that actually have the disease out of the total number of patients with an abnormal test result. In the example of the D-dimer test for venous thrombosis in the chapter on sensitivity and specificity this would be 34 of 50 patients, which gives a positive predictive value of 68%. In other words, of all patients with an abnormal D-dimer result, 68% will have thrombosis and 32% will not (this is not very helpful). The negative predictive value is determined by calculating the proportion of patients with a normal test result and no thrombosis out of the total number of patients with a normal test result. In the example the negative predictive value would be 49/50 = 98%, in other words a normal D-dimer virtually excludes the presence of thrombosis (which may be helpful in clinical practice).

Example

Imagine a biochemist in charge of a clinical chemistry laboratory in a hospital that contains a large gastroenterology department specializing in biliary-pancreatic disease. In order to improve the service to the gastroenterologists the biochemist has recently introduced a novel amylase test that may be helpful in the diagnosis of acute pancreatitis. According to the literature, this new test has a sensitivity of 90% and a specificity of 90%. About 50% of patients in whom there is a clinical suspicion of acute pancreatitis are actually confirmed to have it (with ultrasound, CT scan and a number of other tests). These figures enable calculation of the following positive and negative predictive value of an elevated amylase level for the diagnosis of acute pancreatitis:

	Acute pancreatitis	No acute pancreatitis	
Amylase elevated	45	5	(50)
Amylase normal	5	45	(50)
	(50)	(50)	

Acute pancreatitis is indeed present in 45 out of 50 patients with an elevated amylase level; hence the positive predictive value of an elevated amylase for the diagnosis of acute pancreatitis is 45/50 = 90%. Similarly, 45 patients without pancreatitis have normal amylase levels, giving a negative predictive value of 90% as well. These results are encouraging and it is decided to offer the same amylase test to the local general practitioners. They will occasionally see patients who may have acute pancreatitis. However, the GPs decide that the test is no good for them as they believe that the positive predictive value of the test is only 50% (i.e. no better than tossing a coin). They have calculated this predictive value using the following 2×2 table:

	Acute pancreatitis	No acute pancreatitis	
Amylase elevated	9	9	(18)
Amylase normal	1	81	(82)
	(10)	(90)	

A positive test result (elevated amylase) is present in nine patients with and nine patients without acute pancreatitis, a positive predictive value of 50%. Note that the difference between the two tables is the prevalence of the disease. This is 50% in a gastroenterological referral setting but only 10% in a primary care setting. The difference in prevalence has apparently profound effects on the positive and negative predictive values.

The prevalence of the disease affects the positive and negative predictive value

While the positive and negative predictive values are dependent on the actual prevalence of the disease (as determined by the gold standard), the sensitivity and specificity of the test are independent of the prevalence of the disease. Indeed, in the example in the GP setting, the sensitivity and specificity are both still 90%. In other words, sensitivity and specificity are intrinsic markers for the accuracy of a test, independent of the circumstances. To answer the question whether an abnormal or normal test result is helpful in establishing or excluding the disease, the positive and negative predictive values are probably more relevant, but then the prevalence has to be taken into account. To precisely establish the value of a given diagnostic test in a specific setting the prevalence of the disease in this setting (or the pre-test likelihood) and the predictive value of the test (often expressed as 'likelihood ratio') can be used to calculate the post-test likelihood; if the difference between the pre- and post-test likelihood is large, the diagnostic test will probably yield useful information in this setting (this is covered in more depth in the chapter on likelihood ratios).

Further reading

Jaeschke R, et al. Users guide to the medical literature. VI. How to use an article about a diagnostic test: B. What are the results and will they help me in caring for my patients. JAMA 1994; 271: 703–707.
McGinn T, et al. Clinical prediction guides. Evidence Based Medicine 1998; 3: 5–6.

Related topics of interest

Screening (p. 50); Sensitivity and specificity (p. 90); Likelihood ratios (p. 92).

STRATIFICATION AND MINIMIZATION

Roland M. Valori

In clinical trials the primary purpose of random allocation of patients into experimental groups is to eliminate bias. With other forms of allocation it is possible for bias in the allocation process to make one group systematically different from the other. This difference may influence the outcome of the study. Most randomized trials will include a table of patient characteristics to demonstrate how effective the randomization process has been at dividing patients into similar groups.

While randomization is a very effective way to eliminate bias, it does not guarantee that the experimental groups will be equal for all characteristics that might influence outcome. In fact it is quite possible for the groups to be so different that the outcome of the trial is misleading. This occurred in a trial of azathioprine in primary biliary cirrhosis (*Gastroenterology* 1985; **89:** 1084–1091). The initial result of the trial was that there was no difference between azathioprine and placebo. However, bilirubin is known to be the single most important prognostic factor in primary biliary cirrhosis and the bilirubin levels were significantly higher in the azathioprine-treated patients. Using a Cox multiple regression analysis and adjusting for this imbalance between the two groups, it was concluded that azathioprine did have a statistically and clinically significant effect on outcome, extending survival by 20 months.

Statisticians can usually correct for such imbalances in experimental groups after the study has been done. However, this a relatively clumsy way to do things and many trialists try to make sure that the randomization process allocates patients with important prognostic characteristics equally to each of the experimental groups. This process is called **prognostic stratification** (*Journal of Chronic Disease* 1974; **27:** 365–375).

Prognostic stratification (or stratified block randomization)

The first step in prognostic stratification is to determine which characteristics might affect outcome. Age and sex are obvious examples. Evidence of heart failure in trials of ACE inhibitors after myocardial infarction, or previous venous thrombosis in trials of patients undergoing hip replacement are others. The second step is to rank prognostic factors according to the extent to which they are expected to influence the primary outcome. The third step is for all the subjects to be divided into subgroups according to the highest-ranking factor. These subgroups are further divided according to the next prognostic factor and so on. The final step is random allocation of subjects in each of the subgroups to each of the experimental groups (there may of course be more than two of these).

This process is illustrated in Figure 1. A sample is divided into subgroups according to prognostic factor A (+/−). Each of these subgroups is further divided according to prognostic factor B (+/−). The four resultant groups or 'blocks' are each divided by random allocation to two experimental groups: control and treatment.

In the primary biliary cirrhosis study, prior prognostic stratification for bilirubin would have reduced the chance of imbalance between the study groups and the initial, misleading small difference observed between the groups.

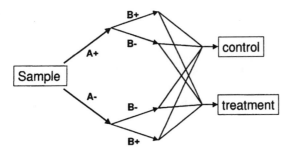

Figure 1. Prognostic stratification for prognostic variables A and B.

It is unusual to see stratification for more than two prognostic factors because further stratification results in a very large and unmanageable number of subgroups. Stratification of two factors yields a minimum of four subgroups (see Figure 1) and three factors, eight. It is important to point out that this procedure is only possible when the differences in the subgroups may have a quantitative effect on the outcome of the trial. If a subgroup exerts a qualitative difference, such as an opposite effect on the outcome, this subgroup is best left out of the study altogether.

Finally, in multi-centre studies it is usual to stratify by centre so that each centre has an equal number in each of the treatment groups.

Minimization

An alternative to stratification prior to randomization is **minimization**. It is possible to make adjustments for imbalance between treatment groups as a trial proceeds. A computer-generated randomization process can be instructed to alter the chances of allocation to one or other groups as the trial proceeds to correct such an imbalance. For example, if too many patients with a particular characteristic have been allocated to the active treatment group the computer can be instructed to weight further allocation in favour of placebo in a ratio of 70:30. As the allocation reaches more equal proportions then the randomization programme can be instructed to revert back to the 50:50 chance of allocation with which it started.

Appraisal tips

If prognostic stratification has been used, try to determine whether the most important prognostic factors have been chosen. Some statisticians regard prognostic stratification as a sophisticated form of window-dressing. They only condone the use of prognostic stratification because they believe the unsophisticated reader might disregard the results of the trial if the experimental groups are not equal, particularly if complicated statistics are used to correct for imbalances, as was done in the azathioprine trial for primary biliary cirrhosis. Beware of studies that do not include a table of important patient characteristics. If there are important differences, try to determine whether an attempt has been made to correct for them in the final analysis of the primary outcome measure. If it has, and if the journal regularly employs statisticians to review their articles, the chances are that it has been done properly and the results of the trial are valid.

Example

In a trial of computer-based decision support (CDSS; *BMJ* 2000; **320:** 686–690) practices were stratified by the type of computer system they were using (in this case EMIS or AAH Meditel). This was done because although the two computer systems had the same CDSS, inevitably there were differences in the way that it interacted with the rest of the computer system. These differences, along with potential differences in the type of practice using a particular computer system, might have affected the way in which the CDSS was used and so needed to be controlled for.

Further reading

Pocock SJ. Methods of randomization. In: *Clinical trials.* Chichester, John Wiley and Sons, 1983; pp. 66–89.

White SJ, Freedman LS. Allocation of patients to treatment groups in a controlled clinical study. *British Journal of Cancer* 1978; **37:** 849–857.

Zelen M. The randomization and stratification of patients in clinical trials. *Journal of Chronic Disease* 1974; **27:** 365–375.

Related topics of interest

Randomized controlled trials (p. 25); Statistical methods (overview) (p. 73); Bias and confounders (p. 101); Subgroup analysis (p. 117).

BIAS AND CONFOUNDERS

Roland M. Valori

Bias refers to errors in study design and execution, and to interpretation and implementation of its results, which systematically influence the eventual outcome for the patient. Bias occurs in both quantitative and qualitative research and it can occur at any stage from conception of a study through to marketing and implementation of its results. Bias can be deliberate or unintentional.

Figure 1 illustrates the relationship of bias to precision and accuracy. The perfect study is one that is both accurate and precise without bias. An accurate study may be imprecise but not biased. A biased study can be precise but still be inaccurate.

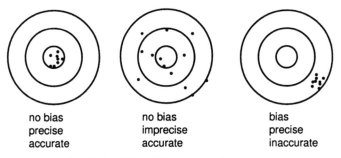

no bias	no bias	bias
precise	imprecise	precise
accurate	accurate	inaccurate

Figure 1. The relationship of bias to precision and accuracy.

Research question

A well-designed study will be constructed around the research question. If the question is biased then the subsequent study will be biased, regardless of its methodological quality. Detecting bias in the formulation of the research question is particularly difficult. However, awareness of this possibility and of the types of biases which occur at this stage of research will considerably improve the chance of detecting them.

Some researchers begin with a strong belief about a particular clinical uncertainty and wittingly or unwittingly formulate the research question in such a way that the outcome of the study is more likely to reinforce their prior beliefs. Such errors can occur as a result of incomplete or deliberately biased assessment of the available literature.

Research questions are more likely to reflect what the investigator regards as important and this may not coincide with the priorities of patients or other clinicians. This is particularly the case for research commissioned by the pharmaceutical industry. Research question bias is not confined to primary research. Questions posed for systematic reviews or meta-analyses may reflect the volume and quality of the available primary research rather than the issues that are important to patients.

Increased awareness of the importance of patient-centred research, and input from patient groups and qualitative research are increasingly influencing the formulation of research questions, thus reducing this type of bias.

Study design

The most common and important biases in study design occur in patient selection and the measurement of outcomes.

Clearly, if patients allocated to control and experimental groups are not similar then differences in outcomes between the two could be due to differences between the groups and not to the intervention they received. It is sometimes possible to predict which factors will affect outcome such as age or sex. However, it is not possible to anticipate all such potentially confounding factors nor to ensure, through a selection process, that they are equally distributed between the groups. Randomization of patients to treatment groups ensures that if there are factors that influence prognosis, they will be evenly distributed between groups whether they are recognized as relevant or not. However, randomization does not guarantee even allocation; it just maximizes the chance of it.

Measurement of outcomes is another important source of bias. Objective outcome measures and blinding both participants and researchers to the allocation group are the main methods for eliminating measurement bias. Hence the term 'double-blind randomized controlled trial'. Clearly it is not always possible (or even desirable) to have objective outcome measures nor to blind both patient and investigator to the allocation group. However, if the study could have been conducted in a double-blind fashion and was not, then it must be regarded with considerable caution. If the study could not have been conducted double-blind with objective outcome measures, then the authors should be expected to discuss in what ways they have guarded against bias.

While randomization is the gold-standard technique for reducing selection bias it is not immune from bias itself.

It is not always possible to do a randomized controlled trial. Avoiding bias in alternative study designs is particularly difficult. Fortunately these biases can be distilled into two questions.

1. Was the selection of cases and controls identical in all regards except the presence of the risk factor being studied?
2. Were measurements on the subjects free from bias?

Statistics

Bias can result from misuse of statistical tests. The most common types of bias are using the wrong test for the data; inferring that there is no difference between treatments when the study is underpowered; and multiple testing.

Peer review and publication bias

High-quality studies that address important clinical questions are generally subject to rigorous and objective peer review and are usually published in a timely fashion in an appropriate journal. However, despite the ascendancy of the randomized controlled trial, the majority of published work is not of high quality and does not always address 'important' questions from the patient's perspective. It is this majority that is subject to peer review and publication bias.

Editors of journals do not always have sufficient expertise to judge whether a submitted article is methodologically sound and frequently ask for help from external peer reviewers. These are usually 'experts' in the field who have a publication record themselves. The reviewing process does not rely totally on objective criteria and is, therefore, subject to bias. It is not difficult to imagine how a research study that does not fit with the reviewer's view on the subject, or with his perception of what is important, may receive a less favourable assessment. Such bias will tend to perpetuate the current view and reject the less orthodox.

Similarly editors may be subject (wittingly or otherwise) to biases and fashions that systematically favour or discriminate against a particular type of research or patterns of results. The best example of this is the bias of a positive result. A study with a positive outcome is much more likely to be published than one with a negative one. Furthermore investigators are more likely to try to publish positive studies than negative ones. If important negative studies are not published, or if they are published after a delay, then meta-analyses can overestimate the true effect of an intervention. There are methods available for detecting publication bias and the pharmaceutical industry is now responding to pressure to release unpublished studies that have not shown positive results. Furthermore, there is now a controlled clinical trials register in the UK which will make tracking of unpublished negative trials much easier.

Dissemination and implementation bias

New evidence is worthless if it is not used and it may be harmful if it is misused. Pharmaceutical companies go to extraordinary lengths to present results of their trials in a favourable light and they occasionally prevent publication of trials. Recently there has been a moratorium on unpublished trials and several large pharmaceutical companies have released a lot of previously unpublished research.

Confounders

Confounders are factors extraneous to the research question that are determinants of the outcome of the study. If they are unevenly distributed between the groups they can lead to bias. A confounder need not be causal; it might be just a correlate of a causal factor. For example, age is associated with a host of disease processes but it is only a marker for underlying biological processes that are causally responsible for these diseases. Similarly, the water pump disconnected by John Snow in Limehouse was not the cause of the cholera, just the conduit that delivered the causal agent.

Procedures for dealing with confounders prior to a study include exclusion, stratified sampling, pairwise matching and randomization. After a study, corrections can be made by using standardization techniques, stratified analysis or multivariate analysis. Prior randomization, whenever possible, is the preferred method of eliminating the effect of confounders.

Appraisal tips

The first step is to identify possible bias or confounders and then make a judgement as to whether they might affect the outcome of the study. If they could, try to determine in what direction they may be influencing the result. If patients are missing from the analysis it is possible to do a worse case sensitivity analysis by allocating each missing patient an unfavourable outcome. If the study retains its clinical and statistical significance then the results are probably valid.

Further reading

Begg CB. Biases in the assessment of diagnostic tests. *Statistics in Medicine* 1987; **6:** 411–423.

Chalmers TC, Celano P, Sacks HS, Smith H. Bias in treatment assignment in controlled trials. *New England Journal of Medicine* 1983; **309:** 1358–1361.

Easterbrook P, *et al.* Publication bias in clinical research. *Lancet* 1991; **337:** 867–872.

Egger M, Davey Smith G. Bias in location and selection of studies. *British Medical Journal* 1998; **316:** 61–66.

Horton R. The less acceptable face of bias. *Lancet* 2000; **356:** 959–960.

Muir Gray JA. *Evidence-based health care. How to make health policy and management decisions.* London, Churchill Livingstone, 1997.

Sackett DL. Bias in analytic research. *Journal of Chronic Disease* 1979; **32:** 51–63.

Related topics of interest

Natural history of disease (p. 1); Randomized controlled trials (p. 25); Sources of information (p. 57); The Cochrane Collaboration (p. 67); Critical appraisal (p. 70); Statistical methods (overview) (p. 73); Subgroup analysis (p. 117).

INTENTION TO TREAT

William S.M. Summerskill

'Intention to treat' (ITT) is the introduction of clinical reality to research trials, by recognizing that, for a variety of reasons, not all patients receive the intended treatment. Patients may deviate from the intended protocol because of misdiagnosis, non-compliance or withdrawal. Using ITT analysis gives a measure of *effectiveness*, a reflection of every-day practice *in vivo*, rather than *efficacy*, the potential impact of an intervention *in vitro*.

Definition

At the heart of a randomized controlled trial is the comparison between intervention and control groups. 'Intention to treat' implies that the analysis of the two groups is on the basis of randomization, so that any difference in outcome is attributable solely to the intervention and no other factors. From the point of randomization onward, an individual is part of the trial, even if in retrospect he/she did not satisfy entry criteria. At randomization it is the investigators' intention that an individual receive treatment/placebo. Although some patients may not receive treatment/placebo, or complete the protocol, they have entered the trial, and must be included in the analysis. Failure to do so, compromises the study design, and biases the findings.

Calculation

A paper's claim of 'intention to treat analysis' must be confirmed by assuring that the numbers 'add up'. Simply stated, all of the participants must be accounted for. The population in each arm of the trial should be the same at randomization and at analysis.

Application

Intention to treat should be considered an entire trial strategy, as a form of 'quality control', rather than just an analytic tool. Because ITT is so unforgiving, its use should improve rigour by emphasizing the importance of accurate diagnosis, obsessive data collection and vigilant follow-up.

ITT is designed for RCTs with hard endpoints, such as survival. In equivalence trials (comparing non-placebo alternative interventions), ITT may reduce the likelihood of disproving the null hypothesis. This also affects crossover trials when participants withdraw after the first intervention.

Interpretation

According to the CONSORT statement (*JAMA* 1996; **276:** 637–639), papers must state whether or not analysis is on the basis of ITT. Trials cannot claim 'intention to treat' if the randomized populations differ from the analyzed populations, unless such exclusions have been explicitly stated and justified prior to randomization. Excluding patients for the following reasons causes bias and is not compatible with ITT:

- Failure to receive or complete treatment/placebo.
- Missing outcome data.
- False inclusions.

Unjustified exclusions

1. *Intervention not started.* If patients have not received an intervention, why should they be included in analysis? In the European Coronary Surgery Study of bypass grafts for stable angina, 768 men with coronary heart disease were randomized between medical and surgical treatment (*Lancet* 1979; **i:** 889–893). Six patients died before receiving surgical treatment and were included in the analysis as deaths for that intervention arm. The trial demonstrated no difference between medical and surgical management, but had the deaths been excluded, surgical intervention would have appeared more favourable. A conclusion that excluded the pre-operative deaths would have been biased because some delays in operating invariable accompany the decision for surgery.

2. *Intervention not completed.* Compliance in drug trials can now be measured and is far less than the 90% claimed. Even among Swiss patients, only one-in-six managed daily compliance for a month (*Statistics in Medicine* 1998; **17:** 251–267). In the future, specific compliance figures may help to appraise the benefit of interventions. At present ITT offers the best solution, as patients in other arms of the trial may be equally poor compliers (as may the parent population, or the individual for whom one is seeking evidence). Exclusion of poor compliers introduces potential bias by undermining the randomization process and selecting for compliance, which may itself be a co-variate for the outcome measure.

3. *Missing data.* Incomplete data is common in clinical trials. The greater the number of missing values, the greater the uncertainty of any conclusions. Various methods are applied to address this problem, but there is no standardized approach. The study can be shortened to use the last complete data set as an end point. Alternatively a sensitivity analysis can be performed comparing the scenarios for different combinations of extreme outcomes.

4. *False inclusions.* If patients are excluded on the grounds of misclassification, then all patients would have to be checked to confirm appropriate classification. A pragmatic approach suggests that some individuals may be misclassified in clinical medicine as in research, and that intention to treat analysis offers the most objective way to acknowledge these individuals when assessing the outcome of specific interventions.

Intention to treat should not be confused with 'per protocol analysis'. In the latter, participants are analyzed according to the intended protocol – and therefore any exceptions to the protocol are excluded.

Further reading

Hollis S, Campbell F. What is meant by intention to treat analysis? Survey of published randomized controlled trials. *BMJ* 1999; **319:** 670–674.

Lewis JA, Machin D. Intention to treat – who should use ITT? *British Journal of Cancer* 1993; **68:** 647–650.

Related topics of interest

Randomized controlled trials (p. 25); Statistical methods (overview) (p. 73); Bias and confounders (p. 101).

THE POWER OF STUDIES

Marcel Levi

In theory, the results of clinical trials are reflections of reality. However, it is possible that any given result of a clinical trial is due to chance alone and does not reflect the real situation. Statistical analysis of results is helpful to demonstrate how large the chance is that a finding is due to chance alone and does not reflect the truth. In biomedical literature, 95% confidence that the result reflects the reality is thought to be acceptable. The certainty that a finding is true is often expressed by calculation of the *P* value. Following the concept of 95% confidence, a *P* value of <0.05 is considered to represent a statistically significant effect. The magnitude of the *P* value does not say anything about the magnitude of the difference between two groups of data, but merely reflects the certainty that the difference is not due to chance alone. However, if no such statistically significant differences are found, this does not necessarily mean that there is no difference between two series of data. It might well be that there is in fact a difference, but that this difference cannot be detected with statistical certainty because of the sample size of the study. The probability that a study falsely rejects the study hypothesis (because the results are not statistically significant), is a function of the power of a study. In other words, the power of a study is the ability of the study to be able to find a lack of difference between two sets of data that is not due to too small a sample size. Typically, a power of 80% is considered to be adequate. Obviously, awareness of the desired power of a study is essential in calculating the sample size needed before it begins.

Example

Cardiac rehabilitation post-myocardial infarction (MI) aims to improve long-term outcome and typically consists of exercise programmes which may or may not be combined with more complex multi-disciplinary interventions. The original trials in this area were generally small and almost all failed to find a significant improvement in mortality with rehabilitation. A power calculation easily explains this inability to detect statistically significant differences in mortality between patients receiving rehabilitation post-MI and control. If we assume that rehabilitation reduces post-MI mortality by 20% (from 5% to 4%) and the desired power is 0.80, we can calculate that we will need at least 6745 patients in each group to be able to detect a statistically significant effect of this magnitude. A smaller effect would require even bigger numbers.

None of the published controlled trials of cardiac rehabilitation included such a large number of patients, which may explain why none of these trials found a significant reduction in mortality.

Power calculations

Ideally, every investigator should perform a sample size calculation in the design phase of studies. Indeed most research ethical committees insist on power calculations in research applications. Important considerations for the calculation are the incidence of the primary outcome parameter in the control group (2% in the example) and the expected reduction by the intervention (50% in the example). This will give a p_1 (proportion of exposure in the study group that undergoes the intervention = 0.01 in the example) and a p_0 (proportion of exposure among controls = 0.02 in the example). Assuming a power (β-value) of 0.80 and a two-sided α-value of 0.05 (level of significance that is usually taken) the required sample size can be calculated using the formula:

$$n \text{ (each group)} = \frac{(p_0^*(1-p_1))+(p_1^*(1-p_0)) * 7.84}{(p1-p0)^2}$$

Following this equation, the power of a study is dependent of the incidence of the outcome parameter, the magnitude of the effect of the intervention and the size of the study population.

Interpreting underpowered data

Based on the above, it is not justified to state that there is no difference between two groups, despite there being no statistically significant difference observed, if the study is insufficiently powered. The only conclusion may be that the design of the study does not permit a definitive conclusion. If there are more studies on the subject that are all underpowered to detect statistically significant results due to their limited sample size, a statistical overview in the form of a meta-analysis may provide a solution.

Further reading

Farrell B. Efficient management of randomized controlled trials: nature or nurture. *BMJ* 1998; **317:** 1236–1239.

Feinstein AR. *Clinical epidemiology: The architecture of clinical research.* WB Saunders Company, Philadelphia, 1985.

Knapp TR. The overemphasis on power analysis. *Nurs Res* 1996; **45:** 379–381.

Related topics of interest

Meta-analyses (p. 19); The *P* value (p. 77).

REPRODUCIBILITY

Marcel Levi

Ideally, two independent observers will find identical results when examining an identical object. Similarly, an observer should find an identical result when examining the same object for a second (or even third etc.) time. However, disagreement often occurs; disagreement between two examiners is termed inter-observer variability, whereas disagreement within one examiner over time is called intra-observer variability. In general, intra-observer variability is usually somewhat less than inter-observer variability. Disagreement over the interpretation of a test not only occurs in research but is also quite common in everyday clinical medicine. Clinicians often disagree with colleagues about the interpretation of patients' histories, physical findings or test results, as indicated in the example.

Quantification of inter- and intra-observer variability

The degree of inter- or intra-observer variability can be calculated simply by dividing the total number of agreements between two examinations over the total number of observations. However, such a calculation does not take into account that there will be agreement based on chance alone. A more precise estimation of variability, which corrects for the expected agreement based on chance alone, is expressed as the *kappa* (κ) value. The *kappa* is the proportion of actual agreement to potential agreement beyond the agreement due to chance alone. To calculate the *kappa*, one should first estimate the agreement expected on the basis of chance. This figure is obviously dependent on the prevalence of a certain test result. For example: if a test result occurs 50% of the time, the alternative test result also occurs 50% of the time, and the agreement expected on the basis of chance is 50%. However, if the prevalence of a test result in both examinations is 70% or even 90%, the per cent agreement expected on the basis of chance alone is 58% and 82%, respectively. The precise per cent agreement to be expected on the basis of chance alone is:

$$\frac{(a1 \times b1) + (a2 \times b2)}{n}$$

where a1 = the percentage of test result (1) by examiner a, a2 = the number of the alternative test result (2) by examiner a, b1 = the percentage of test result (1) by examiner b, b2 = the number of the alternative test result (2) by examiner b, and n = the number of observations. With this figure, it is not difficult to calculate the actual agreement beyond chance (observed agreement minus agreement based on chance alone). Similarly, the potential agreement beyond chance may be calculated (100% minus agreement based on chance alone). The *kappa* value is calculated by taking the ratio of the actual to potential agreement beyond chance.

Example

Assessment of the presence of hepatomegaly is an important feature of physical examination. In a sample of 100 patients with viral lymphadenopathy, one examiner confirms the presence of hepatomegaly in 30 patients. A second examiner establishes the presence of hepatomegaly in 25 patients. Note that the patients that are judged to have hepatomegaly by each of the two examiners are not necessarily the same. Both examiners agree in their judgement 71% of the time. The agreement expected on the basis of chance is:

$$\frac{(30 \times 25) + (70 \times 75)}{100} = 60\%$$

Hence, the actual agreement beyond agreement due to chance alone is 71% − 60% = 11% and the potential agreement beyond chance alone is 100% − 60% = 40%. The kappa value is 11%/40% = 0.28.

Interpretation of the kappa value

How can we interpret this *kappa* value? Some authors have assigned a qualitative classification to various *kappa* values:

kappa	Agreement
0–0.2	slight
0.2–0.4	fair
0.4–0.6	moderate
0.6–0.8	substantial
0.8–1.0	almost perfect

As one can see, the agreement in the assessment of hepatomegaly in our example is only fair using this classification.

Not all test results may be expressed simply in terms of yes or no. Interestingly, calculation of the *kappa* also allows for determining variability at multiple levels of agreement (for example: the liver is normal, 0–5 cm enlarged, or >5 cm enlarged). Since a different opinion as to whether the liver is somewhat more or less than 5 cm enlarged may not be as bad as a divergent opinion on hepatomegaly of >5 cm and a normal liver size, the *kappa* may be weighted for the degree of this disagreement.

Improvement of inter- and intra-observer variability

If one wants to improve variability in the assessment or interpretation of a test result, it is important to realize which factors may play a role in the development of this variability. These may be:

- Examiner-dependent factors (such as inter-individual differences in appreciation of signs, the tendency to interpret signs rather than to observe them, and bias by anticipation of a certain test result),
- Factors that are dependent upon the examined object, caused by natural variation or selective presentation and
- Factors that are dependent on the execution of the examination (including environmental factors or interaction between examiner and examined object).

There are several methods to prevent or minimize the variability of a test result, such as blinding the examiner and standardizing the examination. Development of a simple and standardized scoring system for complicated test results may significantly reduce inter- and intra-observer variability. For example, inter- and intra-observer variability in assessing lung scintigrams for the presence or absence of pulmonary embolism was reduced after introduction of a standardized scoring system using a lung segment reference chart. The inter-observer *kappa* significantly increased from 0.62 in the standard assessment of lung scans to 0.86 when using the standardized method, whereas the *kappa* for intra-observer agreement significantly increased from 0.8 to 1.0.

Further reading

Ingelfinger JA, *et al. Biostatistics in clinical medicine.* 3rd Edition. McGraw-Hill, Inc, New York, 1994.

Lensing AWA, *et al.* Ventilation-perfusion lung scanning and the diagnosis of pulmonary embolism: improvement of observer agreement by the use of a lung segment reference chart. *Thromb Haemostas* 1992; **68**: 245–249.

REGRESSION ANALYSIS

Marcel Levi

Regression is a technique used to express how one value varies depending on the value of another. Regression is used in various ways to establish the relationship between the two variables. In order to understand regression it is necessary to consider a simple equation.

Linear regression

This is the simplest form of regression where the relationship between two values (here x and y) is described by a straight line. A linear regression is usually expressed by the formula:

$$y = a + bx$$

Where *a* is a constant and *b* represents the gradient of the line. If *b* is either greater or less than zero there is a relationship between *x* and *y*, in other words, *y* will increase or decrease with increasing values of *x*. Another term for *b* is the regression coefficient. The value of *a* represents the intercept where *x* equals 0 (see Figure 1).

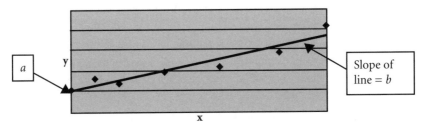

Figure 1.   The graph shows a line which crosses the y axis at *a* and has a gradient *b*.

It should be realized that the assumption of linearity may be justified by real observations but often linearity is used as a convenient summary of data within the range of *x* values that are of interest. When the relationship between two variables is not linear, it may be possible to transform one of the variables (by converting the values to a log scale for example) to achieve linearity in order to perform a regression analysis.

Logistic regression and multiple regression

Logistic regression is a particular form of linear regression that is especially suited to analyse data with a binary outcome, such as death or survival. In addition a binary *x*-value (e.g. smoking or not smoking) can be applied. Logistic regression is often used to assess odds ratios in case–control studies. The use of this type of analysis allows for the correction of potential confounding factors. Multiple regression is a method for using several variables at the same time to improve the estimation of the results.

Using regression in clinical situations

Ingelfinger *et al.* describe six typical clinical implications of regression in biomedical science:

1. Use of regression in disease prevention for example the description of the relation between alcohol intake and liver function, or the relation between the number of cigarettes per day and spirometric parameters.

2. Description of physiology and pathophysiology the relationship between age and renal function or the relation between the creatinine kinase level during acute myocardial infarction and subsequent left ventricular function.

3. Description of disease detection and diagnosis including the phenomenon of regression to the mean, which explains that after an abnormal measurement a subsequent measurement is likely to be more normal.

4. Use of regression to describe treatment effects the relationship between drug dosage and desired or unwanted effects, or the relationship between treatment duration and success in psychotherapy.

5. Regression to predict prognosis for example the number of cytogenetic abnormalities to predict the relapse of acute myelogenous leukaemia or the number of 'pack-years' of smoking as related to the chance of developing an atherosclerotic complication.

6. Regression to describe health care delivery describing the relationship between socio-economic class and the likelihood of having a coronary artery bypass or the relationship between the age of the patient and the length of hospitalization for elective surgery.

Regression analysis may also be useful in other ways:

- to describe the relationship of one variable to another (e.g. to express creatinine clearance as a function of the plasma creatinine level);
- to adjust two sets of variables, in particular when two sets of outcomes (y-values) tend to have different associated x-values (for example to adjust the ejection fraction from echocardiography in a group of patients of varying age, some of whom have diabetes. Both diabetic status and age need to be considered as both will have an independent effect on ejection fraction);
- to forecast a result beyond the range that was actually studied: this is often done in pharmacological research, where plots may predict the effect of very high doses. This is an enterprise fraught with potential problems, however, since there is no evidence, even in the case of linear regression, that the linearity holds true for values below or above the range studied;
- interpretation of a relationship: although a regression analysis can strictly speaking only establish a correlation between two parameters, it may be helpful to formulate hypotheses regarding causality;
- detection of outliers: regression analysis may establish a relationship between abnormal values that on their own would not have been remarkable and may thereby generate novel ideas about disease and treatment.

Example

To establish a relationship between the occurrence of myocardial infarction and the number of cigarettes smoked per day in women, one can collect data on these variables in a sample of subjects. An example of data that may have been collected from such a study is shown in Table 1.

Table 1. Hypothetical relationship between number of cigarettes smoked per day and incidence of myocardial infarction in women

Number of cigarettes/day	Incidence of myocardial infarction/1000
0	0.5
5	0.8
10	0.7
20	1.0
30	1.1
40	1.4
50	2.1

These data can be expressed graphically as shown in Figure 2:

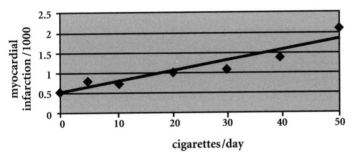

Figure 2. Graph showing relationship between number of cigarettes smoked per day and incidence of myocardial infarction.

The black line on the graph is a 'best fit' line and represents a linear regression through the observed data. The line crosses the y axis at 0.5 (the incidence of MI for a non-smoking woman) and has a slope of 0.035. The formula of the line and hence that of the linear regression is:

$$y = 0.5 + 0.035 * x$$

where y = the number of myocardial infarctions per 1000 persons and x = the number of cigarettes per day.

Inevitably regression analysis can become more complicated than has been described here. For a more advanced consideration of the subject please see further reading below.

Further reading

Altman DG. *Practical statistics for medical research.* Chapman & Hall, London, 1991.

Feinstein AR. *Clinical epidemiology: The architecture of clinical research.* WB Saunders Company, Philadelphia, 1985.

Ingelfinger JA, *et al. Biostatistics in clinical medicine.* 3rd Edition. McGraw-Hill, Inc, New York, 1994.

Willet WC, *et al.* Relative and absolute excess risks of coronary heart disease among women who smoke cigarettes. *N Engl J Med* 1987; **317:** 1303–1308.

Related topics of interest

Determining causation (p. 4); Case–control studies (p. 38).

SUBGROUP ANALYSIS

William S.M. Summerskill

Whereas stratification applies *pre-determined* characteristics, based on criteria that other researchers have found to be of predictive value; sub-group analysis involves a *post hoc* examination of data in search of putative significance. Subgroup analysis is the 'forbidden fruit' of statistical interpretation, because it is irresistibly tempting, but deceptive. Subgroup findings are commonly reported in leading journals. A good critical appraisal will identify subgroup analyses and interpret them with caution.

Quantitative research

Randomized controlled trials are the basis on which interventions are commonly assessed. Given a normal distribution, one in 20 randomized characteristics (covariates) will by chance achieve significance at $p = 0.05$. This is the definition of $p = 0.05$, that there is a 5:100 (1:20) likelihood that the finding may be accounted for by chance alone. Analysis of subgroups carries the same risks of over-interpretation, as does the analysis of multiple outcomes. The risk of a false positive type I error at $p = 0.05$ for one outcome comparison is 5%, for two comparisons it is 10%, for 10 it is 40%, and for 20 it becomes 64%. A survey of 67 trials in *Lancet, NEJM, BMJ* and *JAMA* found the average number of outcomes was 22 (*American Journal of Medicine* 1987; **83:** 545–550). Not surprisingly, the greater the number of outcomes (subgroups) these trials considered, the more 'significant' findings they reported. Type I errors are reduced by adjusting the level of significance, with a lower *P* value threshold in proportion to the number of comparisons performed.

Sample size arises from a 'power calculation' to determine the number of individuals required to detect a change in the primary end-point. Apparent differences in smaller populations, such as sub-groups, may lack 'power' to substantiate their inferences (type I error). The emphasis should be on differences in response to the intervention, not upon differences between groups. For this reason, statistical comparisons are based upon the difference of the intervention upon the separate groups, not upon the results between the groups.

Further uncertainty arises from the fact that an unrelated co-variate achieving significance at randomization is unlikely to influence outcome, whereas a co-variate which is strongly associated with outcome can influence findings even if its distribution between intervention and control groups did not achieve significance.

Because the influence of co-variates may not be known, and could be important, how can one distinguish between significant and spurious findings? First of all, evidence should be based only on those outcome measures specified in the protocol. Second, if a truly compelling, clinically plausible co-variate is identified, it must satisfy interaction tests, and could then be used in a pooled analysis with identical subgroups from other similar studies. If the observation is by chance, it is unlikely to be represented in other studies' subgroups. If the findings are significant, the numerical strength of a meta-analysis will support this. Finally, the substantiated observation should then become the basis of further research to confirm or refute the findings.

When opportunistic subgroup analysis is presented as the principal research finding in a paper, it should be consistent with the overall trial findings. Significant subgroup results in a trial that otherwise failed to demonstrate outcome differences, would raise concerns.

Qualitative research

Subgroup analysis is valued in qualitative research, particularly when generating a hypothesis. If specific information-rich sub-populations are identified in grounded theory studies, they are actively recruited in a data-driven process referred to as *theoretical sampling*.

Example

Counsell *et al.*'s tongue-in-cheek article on DICE therapy for stroke (*BMJ* 1994; **309:** 1677–1681) gives one of the best insights to the principles of evidence-based medicine. In particular, the danger of over-interpreting subgroup analysis is demonstrated when the influence of different colours of dice on outcome are compared. This is compounded if the co-variate of investigator experience (based on rolling dice in a previous trial) and simulated publication bias are also included. Subgroup analysis suggested a 39% reduction in mortality when analysing 'published' trials using green or white dice thrown by an 'experienced' investigator ($p = 0.02$). This is at variance with the overall finding of no treatment benefit ($p > 0.1$). They conclude: 'Don't Ignore Chance Effects' (DICE).

Further reading

Assmann SF, Pocock SJ, Enos LE, Kasten LE. Subgroup analysis and other (mis)uses of baseline data in clinical trials. *Lancet* 2000; **355:** 1064–1069.

Counsell CE, Clarke MJ, Slattery J, Sandercock PAG. The miracle of DICE therapy for stroke: fact or fictional product of subgroup analysis? *BMJ* 1994; **309:** 1677–1681.

Related topics of interest

Outcome measures (p. 7); Stratification and minimization (p. 98); The power of studies (p. 108).

HEALTH STATUS MEASUREMENT

William S.M. Summerskill

Health status measurement, or health-related quality of life (HRQL) measurement, documents the influence of health on a patient's ability to enjoy a fulfilling life. HRQL measurement is becoming a more common component of medical research, since it is implicit (but often empirical) in any clinical decision. Health status measurement provides an evidence base for incorporating patients' experiences and expectations in clinical decisions. It is fundamental to understanding the impact of interventions in terms of well-being and cost.

Theory

Health states are assigned values between 0 (death) and 1 (complete health). Values less than zero describe a health state that is considered worse than death. Health status changes throughout life, and is valued differently by different individuals.

Against what 'yardstick' do individuals measure their health? 'Calman's Gap' defines quality of life inversely as the 'gap' between expectations and achievement. This model allows for changes in expectations as a result of illness or treatment. The smaller the gap, the greater the quality of life (*Journal of Medical Ethics* 1984; **10:** 124–127). Other paradigms include functional and comparative models in relation to that individual's previous health, or the health of his/her peers.

Utilities reflect the population's values rather than objective measurements. Preference-based methods apply judgements about relative health states to derive a score. Non-preference-based approaches focus on the components of health states to provide an aggregate score. The latter method is useful for multiple pathologies or assessing both the benefit of an intervention and its potential side effects.

HRQL measurements can be applied to all domains of mental, physical and social well being, from measuring symptoms to assessing function. Questions regarding possible activities (i.e. *could* you) may overestimate HRQL, while questions referring to actual functional ability (i.e. *can* you) may underestimate health status.

Types of instrument

A review of HRQL measurement in RCTs found 62 different instruments used in 48 trials (*BMJ* 1998; **317:** 1191–1194). Such a variety demonstrates the evolving nature of health status measurement and absence of a single 'gold standard'. Health status measures may be generic (representing universal concepts of function and well-being) or disease-specific. The 36-question short form health survey (SF-36™) is an example of a generic instrument that uses a Likert scale to measure physical and mental health symptoms and function over the previous month (*Medical Care* 1992; **30:** 473–481). Multi-attribute utility scales are specific instruments developed to aid economic analysis, by yielding a single index score, or health status utility.

In addition to rating scales, health status can be measured using *time trade-off* or *standard gamble* techniques. In the former, a patient considers the 'trade' between a shorter length of time in a greater state of health or a longer length of time in a lesser health state. In the latter, the 'gamble' involves determining what probability of success a respondent would accept for an intervention to restore full health if successful, or death if unsuccessful. Patients find time trade-off (TTO) an easier concept than standard gamble (SG). Both methods claim better than 0.75 inter-rater reliability and test–retest coefficients in excess of 0.80, however correlation between the two techniques is low.

Less robust approaches include *magnitude estimation* in which the relative desirability/undesirability between two health states is compared, and *person trade-off* in which the number of people in different health states is adjusted until the resulting product of health state and population is equal between groups.

Different approaches can result in different scores. Overall, standard gamble gives higher utilities than time trade-off, which in turn is higher than rating scales (RS). For example, doctors rated severe angina with utilities of 0.71, 0.53 and 0.35 on SG, TTO and RS respectively (*Social Science and Medicine* 1992; **34:** 559–569).

Discrepancies are attributable to rater experience and attitudes. Standard gamble involves uncertainty and TTO affects lifespan. Values are further influenced by 'anchor points', the reference health state with which comparisons are made. A viral illness takes on different utilities if it is compared with the alternatives of full health (1) or death (0). Furthermore we are used to describing our health in vague colloquial terms such as 'under the weather', not as 0.65.

Health status is defined by individuals. As a result, some researchers have proposed a 'patient-generated index', which provides individuals with an opportunity to identify criteria of personal importance (*Medical Care* 1994; **32:** 1109–1126). By identifying central issues from a patient's perspective, such scales may be useful additions to $n = 1$ trials.

Example

Individuals with the same degree of functional impairment vary in their tolerance of symptoms. Transurethral resection of the prostate (TURP) is considered a quality-of-life enhancing procedure for men with benign prostatic hypertrophy. The resulting improvement in health status depends upon the relative value of prostatic symptoms (urgency, nocturia) compared with those of surgical side effects (incontinence, impotence). A model based on 313 men aged 70 years found that surgery reduced life-expectancy by an average of 1 month, but improved quality of life by 3 months from 120 to 123 months (*JAMA* 1988; **259:** 3010–3017 and 3018–3022). The attractiveness of surgery depends upon the relative impact on quality of life from prostatic symptoms *vs.* the potential side effects of TURP. In response to this finding the authors recommended that the decision to choose surgery for benign prostatic disease should be left up to the patient to make according to his health status preferences.

Interpretation

The principles of measurement are the same for health status measurements as for questionnaires. The method of valuing health or illness needs to be explicit. Who has established the values, how and why? The degree to which instruments provide equal intervals between responses (homoscedasticity), and equal importance between questions will affect the scores and subsequent comparisons. Interpreting HRQL results may be influenced by perspective. Patients, clinicians and administrators can each introduce elements of bias, which must be considered.

Because different instruments measure different aspects of health, the same patient may have different levels of HRQL on different questionnaires. The instrument must be validated for the condition, population (including age), and administration techniques of the particular study; otherwise the findings may not be reliable.

Of special relevance to HRQL measurements are cultural issues that may be lost when an instrument validated in one culture is applied to a different population. This is important for multi-cultural populations in a single country and for large multi-national studies (*Journal of Clinical Epidemiology* 1993; **46:** 1417–1432).

Further reading

Bowling, A. *Measuring Health: A Review of Quality of Life Measurement Scales.* Milton Keynes: Open University Press, 1991.

Brazier J, Deverill M, Green C. A review of the use of health status measures in economic evaluation. *Journal of Health Services Research & Policy* 1999; **4:** 174–184.

Gold MR, Siegel JE, Russell LB, Weinstein MC. *Cost Effectiveness in Health and Medicine.* Oxford, Oxford University Press, 1996.

Related topics of interest

HEALTH ECONOMICS

Roland M. Valori

Until recently the main concern of clinical trials was to establish whether a treatment or other intervention did more good than harm. If a new treatment was found to be effective it was just a matter of time before patients would receive it. With an increasing number of effective treatments available, health care interventions now compete with each other for less resource: we have moved into an era of making choices about health care interventions on the basis of cost as well as efficacy and safety.

Economics is all about **choices** based on value and costs. Health economics is about these choices in the health care setting. The issue now is not 'does it work', but 'is it cost effective?'.

What does cost-effective mean?

Cost-effective is a term that is used rather loosely. Basically it means that a treatment is effective and compares well (in terms of cost) with other treatments that achieve a similar health gain. The important issues are how the costs of an intervention are calculated, and how to put a value on health gain so that interventions can be compared fairly.

1. Calculating costs. Clinical trials increasingly provide cost data to help health professionals and purchasers of health care make choices about resource allocation. Such cost data varies in its sophistication. At one extreme it might only include the direct costs of the intervention and not the costs of administering it. At another extreme it will include the cost of every conceivable impact of the intervention as well as its direct costs. Such costing will include the 'societal costs' such as the effects of time lost from work, and the economic effects of the intervention on carers.

2. Valuing health gain. However sophisticated the measurement of costs it remains hard to compare interventions directly because it is so difficult to place a value on a particular health gain. To overcome this problem health economists have devised a measure that gives a numerical value to health gain called quality-adjusted life years or QALYs.

How are choices made?

Figure 1a illustrates how choices might be made on the balance of costs and health gain. The x-axis represents the health gain of an intervention and the y-axis the costs. To the left of the crossover point the intervention does more harm than good. Below the crossover point the intervention saves money. There are four possible combinations:

1. In the upper left quadrant (A) more harm than good is done and the intervention costs more. Clearly this intervention should not be implemented.
2. In the lower right quadrant (D) there is a health gain and the intervention saves money. This intervention should clearly be implemented.
3. In the left lower quadrant (C) more harm than good is done but the costs are less. Depending on the degree of harm this intervention may be implemented if this

frees up sufficient resource for a treatment with a health gain that will offset the unwanted effects done with the money-saving intervention. In practice it is unusual for such an intervention to be implemented.

4. The upper right quadrant (B) is the most common situation: there is a health gain but it costs more to implement the treatment.

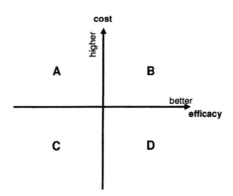

Figure 1a. Comparing costs and efficacy.

*1. **Willingness to pay.*** Figure 1b illustrates the concept of willingness to pay. A line has been drawn through the intersection of cost and efficacy in the 'uncertainty' quadrants (B and C). In quadrant B interventions that fall below the line are relatively efficacious for little cost and those above it relatively expensive for little gain. The angle of this line can be changed so that more or fewer interventions fall below it. This is called the willingness to pay line. The steeper the line the greater the willingness to pay for the intervention (as there is more chance the intervention will appear below the line and vice versa).

The willingness to pay for an intervention depends on the perspective of the individual or group. For example, politicians and the general public might be more willing to pay for investment in coronary artery by-pass grafts or special care baby units.

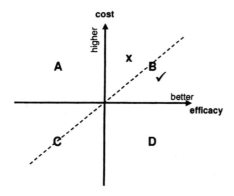

Figure 1b. Willingness to pay.

Conversely they might be less willing to pay for drug rehabilitation units or in-vitro fertilization.

2. Making choices. It can be seen that health economics is not just about costs of health care but also about the value attached to a health gain or the willingness to pay. This value might be perceived differently by different stakeholders such as the public, doctors, other health professionals, purchasers of health care and politicians. Hitherto, doctors have had a major influence on how health care resource has been allocated. The NHS plan is attempting to redress the balance of power, to give the consumers of health care and other health professionals greater say in resource allocation decisions.

Methods of economic analysis

1. Cost description. There is no comparison of treatments or outcomes in this type of analysis, just a description of costs.

2. Cost analysis. In this type of study there is a comparison of costs between treatments but no examination of outcomes.

3. Cost-minimization study. This study compares the costs of different treatments but it assumes that the clinical outcomes in the two groups are identical.

4. Cost-effectiveness analysis. In this analysis there is a comparison between alternative treatments or interventions. The measurement of outcomes is in natural units such as life-years gained, pain-free days, percentage reduction in cardiac events. The result of the study is expressed as a ratio of change in costs to change in effect (the natural units). For example the result of an intervention for acute coronary syndrome might be expressed as £1,000 per myocardial infarction prevented.

5. Cost–utility analysis. This is similar to the cost-effectiveness analysis. The difference is that the clinical outcome is expressed in terms of quality and/or quantity of life. The measurement is usually made in terms of quality-adjusted life years (QALYs). This analysis reduces the clinical outcome to a single currency or unit so that interventions for different conditions can be compared more easily.

6. Cost–benefit analysis. In this type of study alternative interventions are compared but the clinical outcomes are given a monetary valuation. There is then a direct comparison between costs (of the intervention) and the benefits, expressed in monetary value. This type of study is unusual in health care research because of the difficulty in attaching a monetary value to all aspects of a health gain.

Appraisal tips for an economic evaluation

1. Determine whether a true comparison was made between interventions and how strong the study design was (e.g. was it a randomized comparison?).
2. Is it possible to determine exactly what has happened to whom and when?
3. Decide whether all possible outcomes of the interventions have been determined. These should include patient-centred outcomes such as quality-of-life measures, time lost from work, and time spent travelling to and from the hospital.

4. Determine whether all possible health care costs were considered and valued correctly. For example were costs of follow-up in primary care included and were non-health care costs considered?
5. Was a sensitivity analysis (see below) performed on these costs?
6. Were costs adjusted for differential timing (discounting costs)? A cost incurred 'up front' costs more than one occurring months or years later.
7. In the event that an intervention was better but costs more, was there discussion of the possible 'willingness to pay' of different stakeholders – patients, health professionals, purchasers and politicians?

Example

This randomized controlled trial (*BMJ* 1998; **317:** 103–110) compared clinical and economic outcomes of laparoscopic and open hernia repair in 400 patients fit for general anaesthesia. The laparoscopic technique resulted in more short-term pain but better long-term pain control and a reduction in time to return to work. Quality-of-life questionnaire scores (SF-36) indicated patients preferred the laparoscopic technique. There were more minor complications in the open repair group. Costs of laparoscopic repair were £335 greater than open repair (CI: £228–441).

Surgical trials are not easy to conduct because the outcomes cannot be assessed in a blinded fashion, because operations are less predictable interventions than drugs and because most operations are insufficiently frequently performed. Therefore this trial of hernia repair has done well to include an economic analysis as well as a comparison of clinical and patient-centred outcomes.

There is a clear description of how costs were derived and it appears that most Health Service costs were accounted for. Sensitivity analysis was performed to provide an estimate of costs according to whether reusable or 'largely disposable' equipment was used, and for different 'hotel' costs. Reusable equipment abolished the difference in costs, largely disposable equipment accentuated it, and hotel costs did not change the difference between the groups. There was no assessment of societal costs such as the cost of delayed return to work or the costs to carers at home. No adjustments were made for multiple comparisons.

This is a fairly typical **cost-effectiveness analysis** showing how an intervention with an improved clinical outcome (laparoscopic hernia repair) was associated with greater expense (quadrant B Figure 1a). Theoretically a **cost–utility analysis** (applying a QALY to the health gain) would enable local health purchasers to compare this intervention with others in order to help them decide whether they were willing to pay for it. This willingness-to-pay decision (the gradient of the dotted line in Figure 1b) will be influenced by political considerations:

- hernia operations clog up waiting lists;
- more costly operations lead to longer waiting lists because fewer can be done;
- waiting lists are a political priority, therefore politicians will not be willing to pay for the preferred option;
- the willingness to pay gradient (Figure 1b) will be shallow.

Further reading

Department of Epidemiology, Mcmaster University. How to read clinical journals: VII. To understand an economic evaluation (part B). *Canadian Medical Association Journal* 1984; **130:** 1542–1549.

Drummond MF, Stoddart GL, Torrance GA. *Methods for the economic evaluation of health care programmes.* Oxford, Oxford University Press, 1987.

Lockett T. *Health economics for the uninitiated.* Oxford and New York, Radcliffe Medical Press, 1996.

Mooney G. *Key issues in health economics.* Hemel Hempstead, Harvester Wheatsheaf, 1994.

Related topics of interest

QALYs

William S.M. Summerskill

This chapter introduces a patient-based econometric strategy for comparing medical interventions, the quality-adjusted life-year (QALY). QALYs are the product of life expectancy combined with utility. Calculations incorporate the desirability of a specific health state with the time spent in that health state. In this manner evolving conditions can be considered, by using the sum of each constituent health state and its duration.

Figure 1 depicts different health states: perfect health (1a), unchanging mediocrity (1b), gradual deterioration (1c) and fluctuating health (1d). Although life expectancy varies from 11 to 20 years, the sum of each health scenario and the time spent in that health state is 11 QALYs.

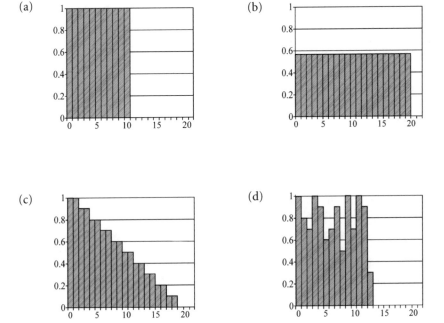

Figure 1. The shaded area in each figure represents 11 QALYs spread over 10–20 years (x axis).

Application

Because they are not disease- or treatment-specific, QALYs can be used to compare outcomes between different conditions to enlighten medical decisions. In cost–utility analysis, the cost/QALY yields a figure for financial decisions. The United States Panel on Cost-Effectiveness in Health and Medicine has recommended the use of QALYs for cost-effectiveness analyses, a decision which will increase reporting of this measure.

Methodological issues

Like a meta-analysis, the comparison of QALYs expects homogeneity. This can only be obtained if QALYs are calculated in a standardized manner. The central issues are 'who' determines the value of a health state and 'how' is this measured.

Health states may be valued differently by health professionals, by those in that health state, or by the community at large. To standardize comparisons, the Panel recommends that relative health-state values are based on community-preferences, i.e. they would reflect the general population's preference for a specific health state.

Any methods used for health status measurement, can be adapted to calculate the quality of different health states. Because of variability, the panel recommends that results based on rating scales should be compared with results obtained from *time trade-off* and *standard gamble*, as these measures are more reliable.

Controversy

Proponents of QALYs cite the combination of quality and length of life, incorporation of patient-preference, use of evidence-based medicine, and ability to compare cost-effectiveness between competing priorities. To many, QALYs provide an easily understood method for maximizing the health gain from available resources.

Critics point out that QALYs do not distinguish between health 'needs' and 'preferences'. The value placed on a health state differs depending on whether an individual is likely to experience that health state or not, and may also change once in a new health state. The concept discriminates against disabled people, as an intervention for an unrelated condition will not restore these individuals to a QALY of 1. It is also 'ageist', since the elderly will have less average life-expectancy.

Health care users with a specific illness rate their quality of life differently than the general public does. When asked to rate hypothetical disease states, respondents exhibit prejudices based on previous disease experience. This undermines the concept of equality between QALYs.

QALYs are designed for chronic conditions and become expensive when applied to acute illness. Because QALYs are based on 1 year as a unit of time, the shorter the duration of health gain, the more costly it becomes. An extreme example is having dental root canal work without a local anaesthetic. This would be painful, perhaps attracting a utility of 0.1. An increase of 0.9 would restore the individual to perfect health (QALY=1) for the 1 hour of the procedure. What would the extra 0.9 QALY for 1 hour be worth? An additional 0.9 QALY for 1 hour represents $\frac{0.9}{365 \times 24} = 0.0001$ QALY for a year. Using the customary ceiling of US $40 000 per QALY, the amount available for a local anaesthetic would be: $40,000 \times 0.0001 = \$4$ (*Health Economics* 2000; **9**: 177–180).

Similar concepts

Small health gains can be expressed as quality-adjusted life-months. The concept of quality *vs.* length of life is also addressed by disability-adjusted life-years (DALYs), healthy life-years (HeaLYs), years of healthy life (YHL), and years of healthy life lost (YHLL).

Interpretation

Before considering QALYs, one must be satisfied that the efficacy and the costings of the intervention are themselves current, evidence-based and appropriate to the population under consideration. QALY calculations must be explicit and address the above methodological issues.

International comparisons reflect differing values for health states between cultures. A study of 14 countries found that HIV infection was ranked as less of a disability in Japan or the United Kingdom than in Egypt, where it was considered the most disabling condition (*Lancet* 1999; **354**: 111–115). There are also socio-economic factors that mitigate or exacerbate the effect of disease states for individuals. For instance, those with co-morbidity will not be restored to perfect health by successful treatment of just one condition. Ignoring the presence of co-morbidity in a population underestimates the cost per QALY for that population.

QALYs are traditionally calculated for chronic conditions, which are not comparable to acute illnesses.

Papers should include a sensitivity analysis, to demonstrate the effect of variations in clinical outcome and costs.

Example

A meta-analysis of 3920 women aged over 50 years with breast cancer involving lymph nodes compared tamoxifen alone with tamoxifen and chemotherapy. The tamoxifen and chemotherapy group gained a non-significant mean 5½ months symptom-free survival and 2 months overall survival in return for chemotherapy lasting between 2 and 24 months. Using hypothetical values, quality of life was lower during the months of chemotherapy, so that overall, the investigators found no difference in quality-adjusted survival time between the two groups at 7 years (*Lancet* 1996; **347**: 1066–1071).

Further reading

Neumann PJ, Zinner DE, Wright JC. Are methods for estimating QALYs in cost-effectiveness analyses improving? *Medical Decision Making* 1997; **17**: 402–408.

Related topics of interest

Outcome measures (p. 7); Health status measurement (p. 119); Health economics (p. 122).

SAMPLING AND APPLICABILITY

Roland M. Valori

The term applicability refers to the extent to which the results of a study are relevant to, or can be applied in, clinical settings other than that of the study. There are two components of applicability to think of when appraising a study: how biologically similar the patients are; and whether the process of the intervention can be replicated. The way the patients have been sampled will tell you how biologically applicable the study is, and details of the intervention and the setting will determine the process applicability.

Sampling

Sampling refers to the means by which the subjects for the study were selected and then recruited. The selection process is made on the basis of inclusion and exclusion criteria. These criteria define the sample. The table of patient characteristics gives an indication of how successful the sampling process has been.

1. Signal to noise ratio. Very strict criteria provide a homogeneous sample that will exhibit less variation ('noise') in the outcome measures when compared to a sample assembled with more lax criteria. With less variation there is a higher signal to noise ratio and a smaller sample size is needed. However, the results of a study with tight entry criteria will apply to fewer people than with those from a study with less strict selection criteria.

2. Generalizability. It can be seen that investigators are faced with a dilemma when designing studies. On the one hand they wish to minimize the numbers of patients that need to be recruited into the study, and on the other they desire the results to be applicable to as many patients in as many health care settings as possible. The extent of this applicability determines the **generalizability** of a study.

Inevitably there is a compromise and investigators usually use stricter criteria because studies with large numbers of patients are extremely difficult to do. The stricter the entry criteria, the greater the need to determine whether the sample is applicable in one's own population. Some investigators have advocated very large simple trials that are generalizable to most health care settings. However, it is clear that some clinical questions can only be answered with small trials because not all illnesses are common.

3. Applicability. When determining applicability for a particular patient it is worth asking whether the patient would have fitted the entry criteria and therefore have been eligible for randomization. If so, then the results of the study are likely to be applicable to that patient. If not, then you should determine how well the entry criteria fit the patient, and then ask whether any useful information can be gleaned from this study to help with the management of that patient. The alternative is to look for another study with entry criteria that are more suited to your patient.

Inclusion and exclusion criteria define the sample but not every patient who fits these criteria will actually end up in the study. This does not matter if the reasons for not being entered are unlikely to affect the outcome of the intervention, but sometimes they will be likely to do so. Things to watch out for are studies that do not record patients eligible for randomization, those with a high non-inclusion rate and those with unequal groups after randomization.

Figure 1 illustrates the concept of applicability. The diagram represents use of anticoagulation in atrial fibrillation to prevent stroke. The study sample will only represent a proportion of all patients with atrial fibrillation. Patients may have been excluded on the basis of age, presence of heart failure, valvular lesions etc. Our own sample may fit some (group A) but not all (group B) of the selection criteria. The results of the trial will be applicable to those in group A but not necessarily to those in group B. The main difference between the two groups might lie in the ages of the patients in each. This difference may be clinically important, because we might expect older patients to benefit more but also experience more harmful effects of treatment.

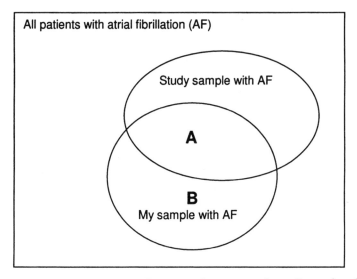

Figure 1. Venn diagram illustrating the concept of sampling and applicability.

If many patients are not being entered it means that either the patients or the investigators feel uncomfortable with allocation to one or other group. This may lead to systematic bias. For example, there may be factors outside the inclusion and exclusion criteria of which the investigator is aware, which make him decide to omit the patient from the study. Likewise, particular patients may not wish to be randomized, or may have a strong preference after randomization for being included in the other group, and then drop out. For this reason it is recommended that randomization should occur as late as possible in the recruitment process.

4. Process. Once the biological applicability has been determined, the next step is to decide whether the intervention can be replicated. The intervention may require expensive medication, particular surgical expertise, special monitoring facilities or community back-up services that are not available in some health care settings. It may not be apparent from the publication that other factors may be needed to replicate it, particularly things that are impossible to measure such as the enthusiasm, drive and ambition of the investigators. Thus it is important to understand how much the intervention will cost and what processes are required to replicate it before planning to implement it.

Worked example

A study by Sharpe *et al.* investigated the efficacy of cognitive behaviour therapy (CBT) for patients with chronic fatigue syndrome (*BMJ* 1996; **312**: 22–26.). Sixty patients were randomized to receive 16 weekly sessions of CBT or their usual medical treatment. There was a 47% difference in response rates between the groups, suggesting that only two patients would need to be treated with CBT to achieve one favourable outcome.

The inclusion and exclusion criteria were quite explicit therefore it would not be difficult to determine whether one's own patient could have been recruited into the study. The intervention is well described and referenced and should therefore be reproducible. An important part of the study was the determination of its acceptability to patients (which it was). However, there is no indication of the costs (and savings) of the intervention, and thus it may be difficult to persuade purchasers that it should be implemented.

The patients included in this trial were recruited from referrals to a secondary care infectious disease clinic in Oxford. Not many hospitals have an infectious disease clinic and Oxford, with a large academic and middle class population, is unique. Therefore, despite the explicit entry criteria it is difficult to know whether this study will be applicable to one's own setting. It is not generalizable to many other clinical settings, particularly primary care, where an effective intervention for chronic fatigue would be most useful.

The next step to address this important question would be to perform a cost-effectiveness study in primary care of CBT for chronic fatigue syndrome with clinical outcomes that are specifically patient-centred.

Further reading

Altman DG, Bland JM. Generalization and extrapolation. *BMJ* 1998; **317**: 409–410.

Guyatt GH, Jaeschke RZ, Cook DJ. Applying the results of clinical trials to individual patients. *ACP Journal Club* **122**: A12–13.

Guyatt GH, Haynes RB, Jaeschke RZ, *et al.* Users' guide to the medical literature: XXV. Evidence-based medicine: principles for applying the users' guides to patient care. *JAMA* 2000; **284**: 1290–1296.

Related topics of interest

Randomized controlled trials (p. 25); Cohort studies (p. 33); Critical appraisal (p. 70); Bias and confounders (p. 101); The power of studies (p. 108); Guidelines (p. 136); Improving professional practice (p. 142).

AUDIT

Dermot P.B. McGovern

The process of audit is ubiquitous within the NHS and it is impossible to escape its reaches. Audit does not strictly fall under the remit of EBM, but together with EBM it is an integral part of clinical governance and, without exception, every practising doctor within the UK should be regularly auditing his or her performance.

The audit cycle as a process has been well documented and is summarized in Figure 1. There are a number of stages in the audit cycle:

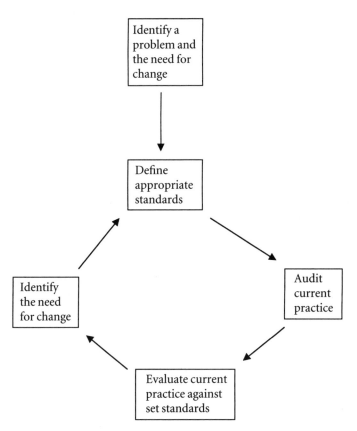

Figure 1. The audit cycle (spiral).

1. Identification of potential clinical failings/problems.
2. Setting of appropriate standards of care.
3. Evaluation (audit) of current practice.
4. Comparison of results (3) against set standards (2).
5. Identify the need and process for change of practice.
6. Re-evaluation of current practice (3).

There can and should be an intricate relationship between audit and EBM as EBM can 'inform' the audit cycle at every stage:

1. *Identification of problems.* Potential problems in practice can be identified from within (i.e. reading an article that highlights a deficiency in current practice) or in a 'top down' fashion (via a directive from an organization such as the National Institute for Clinical Excellence (NICE) or a local opinion leader). In fact this step is 'pure EBM' as identification of a problem should inevitably lead to:

- The construction of a clinical question.
- A search for studies providing answers to the question.
- Critical appraisal of identified studies.
- The implementation of evidence.

2. *Setting standards.* Standards are set as a result of the evidence found from step 1. Knowledge of EBM may also help the auditors set appropriate outcome measures that are achievable and that can be reliably evaluated.

3. *Audit of practice.* Reliable methods of data collection are important for an accurate evaluation of current practice.

4. *Comparison.* A basic understanding of the meaning and use of statistical analysis may be relevant for this part of the audit cycle.

5. *Implementing change.* Healthcare environments are notoriously difficult settings in which to implement change. There is some evidence, however, about successful and unsuccessful methods used to implement change and an excellent, if depressing, review of this subject is the 'No magic bullets' review by Andrew Oxman (see Further reading). This is well worth reading for anyone who may have to change his/her own (or someone else's) practice. There are a number of ways of influencing healthcare professionals' behaviour including the use of guidelines, opinion leaders, near patient reminders etc. and the critical appraisal process can identify which of these is most applicable to the particular setting in question.

6. *Re-audit.* This EBM 'informed' audit process should result in an (upward!) audit spiral rather than an audit cycle (Unfortunately most audits do not even complete the cycle and are in fact audit semi-circles!). Thus audit can show the benefit of EBM through demonstrating improved patient care, thereby actually showing healthcare professionals the benefit of their hard work.

Audit also allows clinicians to obtain evidence about their own practice. This will become increasingly important in:

- Identifying and evaluating poorly performing doctors. Health watchdogs will expect all practitioners to regularly audit their own (and each other's) work.
- Providing true informed consent for patients undergoing procedures. Audit provides ideal data to inform patients of individual practitioner's success and complication rates as part of the consent process.
- Production of the controversial 'league tables' allowing consumers to compare health outcomes in different areas.

Audit can either be a process of self-review (**self audit**) or external review (**peer audit**). Self-audit has the advantages of being cheaper and non-threatening but it may be a less rigorous process, which may be a problem in the current climate of doubts over the validity of self-regulation. Peer audit involves auditors from outside the immediate group evaluating practice. This is certainly more threatening, but may be a more rigorous process. The Commission for Health Improvement (CHImp or CHI) recently set up by the UK government will perform external audit on hospitals, departments, practices or even individual doctors whose practice is providing concern. Anonymous external audit already exists within the NHS including the audits of Perioperative deaths and Maternal and Perinatal deaths.

Example (Audit of care of patients with epilepsy in General Practice. *BJGP* 1996; 46: 731–734)

This study is an excellent example of audit in practice. It describes two rounds of audit of the care of patients with epilepsy in two large practices in Norfolk. The first audit cycle showed 83% of patients had been seen at least once in the previous year, seizure frequency had been recorded in 51% and 63% were taking no more than two medications. These results were presented to the GPs concerned and discussion of how to improve them took place. The evaluation was repeated 22 months later showing 95% of patients seen within the last year, 93% with seizure frequency recorded and 63% on no more than two medications. No formal statistics were done but the results show a definite improvement in two out of three criteria. In an ideal world re-audits are done at regular intervals although this rarely happens in practice.

Further reading

Oxman AD, Thomson MA, Davis DA, Haynes RB. No magic bullets: a systematic review of 102 trials of interventions to improve professional practice. *CMAJ* 1995; **153**(10): 1423–1431.

Related topics of interest

Outcome measures (p. 7); Formulating clinical questions (p. 10); Guidelines (p. 136).

GUIDELINES

William S.M. Summerskill

The National Institute for Clinical Excellence (NICE) defines guidelines as 'systematically developed statements to help health professionals and patients make the best decisions about the most appropriate health care in particular circumstances'. In this context guidelines have the potential to make practice more efficient and more effective. To realize this aim, clinical practice guidelines (CPGs) must incorporate evidence in their design and implementation.

Design

Guidelines are more likely to succeed when they:

- Involve users in their formulation.
- Are based on explicit evidence.
- Complement current medical practice.
- Improve patient care.
- Are presented clearly.
- Are implemented actively.

Guidelines should be implemented with an evaluation programme to assess their impact.

Citations can be found to support almost any medical view/opinion. As demonstrated elsewhere in this book, a journal reference is not synonymous with evidence. Similarly with guidelines, the clinician is interested not only in the integrity of the chosen references, but also in the process of selecting the articles on which a guideline is based. Guideline recommendations should state whether they are based directly on grade A evidence or extrapolated from grade C evidence, etc. Guideline users must satisfy themselves that a systematic review of published and unpublished studies has been undertaken with explicit inclusion criteria, and that the recommendations are grounded in evidence.

Involving the target 'users' in guideline design keeps the process focused on the intended clinical setting. This process improves the sense of user 'ownership', and enhances uptake of CPGs. A balance must be struck between locally generated guidelines, which are more likely to be used, and nationally generated guidelines, which are more likely to reflect evidence-based practice.

Uptake is improved when guidelines are implemented actively. 'Mail shot' recommendations do not change practice. Guidelines are most effectively introduced by multiple methods, including academic outreach, audit and financial support to address the costs of changing practice.

Criticism

Guidelines have been perceived as inflexible 'cookbooks', making it difficult for practitioners to translate trial data to individual patients. The more a clinician knows about a patient, the more individual he or she becomes. This is particularly true in primary care, where guidelines regarding the management of hypertension may not include blood pressure treatments for patients with co-morbidity, erratic lifestyles, or from certain ethnic backgrounds. In these situations, the evidence from well-prepared guidelines are just that: guidance along the lines of best clinical practice.

Example

The National Service Framework for Coronary Heart Disease (London, HMSO: 2000) incorporates evidence at all stages of design and implementation. The 40-member external reference group involved many stakeholders, including GPs, cardiologists, nurses, patient representatives and public health officials. Evidence for blood pressure control and anti-thrombotic treatment came directly from meta-analyses; recommendations for lipid management and β-blockers (after a heart attack) came from RCTs. All are grade A recommendations, which consolidate 'best practice' and improve patient outcomes.

Evidence also directs the implementation process. The NSF is intended to be an example of how multiple evidence-based strategies are used to implement a guideline. Stakeholders participated in the design, ensuring wide ownership of standards. Staff recognized 'skills gaps' and were involved in identifying barriers and opportunities for change. Strategies for behaviour change and incentives for changes were used to implement new procedures. The process was further supported with education, training and new information technology. An annual audit programme will monitor both the process and outcome of CHD care.

Medical behaviour

Guidelines are intended to change behaviour, which explains many of the variables influencing guideline use described above. Doctors change their behaviour cautiously, as a group, rather than as individuals. Peer performance provides a great influence. In this context, CPGs can act like a catalyst, promoting the rate of change.

Medico-legal implications

Some experts believe that guidelines could reduce malpractice litigation by standardizing medical practice. In the United States, CPGs have been used both as inculpatory evidence (plaintiffs) and exculpatory evidence (defendants). They also influence a lawyer's decision to go to court or to settle claims (*Annals of Internal Medicine* 1995; **122:** 450–455).

Assessment

The effectiveness of guidelines remains controversial. Guidelines influence the *process* of care, but do not always exert a measurable effect on the *outcome* of care. CPGs which follow the above criteria appear more likely to be effective at implementing change than those which do not use an evidence-based approach. One reason for the difficulty in measuring impact is their role as 'catalyst'. Guidelines are not introducing, but accelerating the implementation of practice principles. Therefore, it can be difficult to identify the net change attributable to guidelines against the secular drift of changing practice.

The challenge for the National Service Framework is raised by the WHO *MONICA* study: 'is the decline of CHD mortality in wealthy countries attributable to secondary prevention, or other lifestyle changes?' (*Lancet* 2000; **355**: 688–700). This is an important issue to consider, as guidelines are expensive to produce, and their development and implementation costs must be considered in parallel with the cost implications of the guideline intervention.

Further reading

Grimshaw JM, Russell IT. Effect of clinical guidelines on medical practice: a systematic review of rigorous evaluations. *Lancet* 1993; **342:** 1317–1322.

Grol R. Implementing guidelines in general practice care. *Quality in Health Care* 1992; **1:** 184–191.

Related topics of interest

Natural history of disease (p. 1); Hierarchy of evidence (p. 13); Critical appraisal (p. 70); Improving professional practice (p. 142); Limitations of EBM (p. 148).

DECISION ANALYSIS

Marcel Levi

There are very few clinical decisions that can be regarded as simply 'black and white' decisions and the majority of clinical decisions contain a degree of uncertainty. These decisions are usually made after balancing the possible outcomes (both good and bad) that may occur as a result of that decision and also the chances of those outcomes occurring. Even more uncertainty is introduced when decisions that may have variable consequences or involve multiple steps are considered. In this situation 'decision trees' can be constructed to simplify the process. Decision trees can be made for virtually any clinical situation and to a certain degree this is the process that clinicians intuitively use when making decisions about patients' care.

Construction of a decision tree requires detailed information on the chances of the various outcomes occurring following implementation of any decision about clinical care. In addition, it is also necessary to know the sensitivity and specificity of diagnostic tests or the efficacy and safety of the various treatment strategies. A utility (value in terms of quality of life) has to be assigned to each potential outcome. This is highly subjective by definition as no two people will assign precisely the same utility to a given outcome. In an ideal situation, the patient should have an input into the decision-making process by discussing the utility that he or she places on each possible outcome. The expected utility for each branch of the decision tree (based on the estimated utility of the outcome and the probability that this will occur) can be calculated and hence the most optimal treatment strategy may be chosen (see example).

According to Sacket *et al.*, the construction and implementation of a decision tree requires the following six steps:

1. The creation of a tree that stems from the clinical decision and all the possible relevant outcomes;
2. The assignment of probability to each of the outcomes that stem from the decision and calculation of the probabilities of each of the most distal branches (i.e. the probability of each of the potential outcomes) by combining the individual step-wise probabilities;
3. The assignment of utilities (worth to the patient) to each of the outcomes;
4. Multiplication of the probability of each outcome with the utility of this outcome;
5. Choose the option with the highest expected utility;
6. Assess the effect of changes in the probabilities and the utilities within the decision tree.

Example

A patient with symptomatic gastro-oesophageal reflux disease wants to discuss his treatment options with you. He is concerned at the possibility of life-long treatment with proton pump inhibitors. He has heard from a friend that surgery may also be effective, although he understands that there are risks associated with surgery. A literature search reveals that chronic proton pump inhibitor therapy is effective in 90% of cases. Surgery (i.e. a Nissen fundoplication) is equally effective and, if successful, may obviate the need for chronic medication. However, this surgery is associated with a number of complications, including abdominal bloating, dysphagia and an inability to belch. According to the literature the chance of such complications is estimated to be 20%. Figure 1 shows the relevant decision tree analysis for this clinical problem. The chance of each of the possible outcomes stems from the knowledge of these probabilities. For example, the chance of having no symptoms following surgery (90%) but a complication (20% of surgical cases) is 0.18 (i.e. 0.9×0.2) and the chance of having continuing symptoms with medical treatment is 10% (0.1).

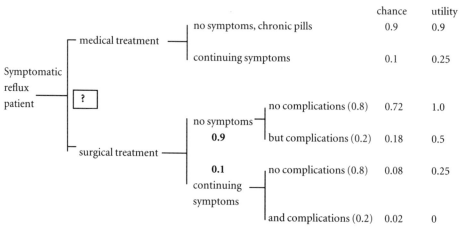

Figure 1. Decision tree analysis of the potential outcomes of medical versus surgical management of gastro-oesophageal reflux disease.

The utilities that are assigned to each of the outcomes are very subjective and should be based on patient preferences where possible. According to the utilities assigned in this example, successful surgery without complications is the best outcome (utility 1.0) and surgery with a bad outcome and complications the worst outcome (utility 0). Successful medical treatment (but chronic medication) is given a utility of 0.9, whereas successful (in terms of symptom control) surgery, but with complications, is assigned a utility of 0.5. The utility of unsuccessful, but uncomplicated, surgery or failed medical treatment is estimated at 0.25. Multiplying the probability with the utility for each outcome allows all resulting expected utilities per branch that stem from the initial decision to be added together. In this example:

- The expected utility of successful medical treatment (0.9×0.9) and unsuccessful medical treatment (0.1×0.25) add up to **0.835**.
- The four possible outcomes of surgery, i.e. 0.72 (0.72×1), 0.09 (0.18×0.5), 0.02 (0.08×0.25) and 0 (0.02×0) add up to **0.83**.

The conclusion is that the overall outcome of medical treatment is likely to be better ($0.835 > 0.83$) than the outcome of surgery.

This example clearly illustrates that precise estimates of probability and utilities are required in order to develop a decision tree. The utilities have a fundamental effect on the outcome of the decision analysis. For example, if this patient felt that taking medication on a long-term basis would significantly impair their quality of life then the utility of successful medical treatment may have been lower, let's say 0.8. If this were the case, surgical treatment would have been the preferred option.

Decision tree analysis allows clinicians to make such calculations in conjunction with their patients and also enables clinicians to tailor the utilities (and probabilities) according to the preferences (and fitness) of the individual patient. Quality-of-life-based research may give us more objective data on which to base these utility values but patient preference should always play a significant role as no two patients will have the same utilities for a given decision. Additionally, decision tree analyses can be adapted to include local complication/success rates again illustrating the flexibility of this technique.

In the example above a therapeutic dilemma was illustrated. Similarly, the choice for a diagnostic strategy may be the subject of a decision analysis, in which case, the test characteristics (i.e. sensitivity and specificity) will determine the chances of each outcome (true or false positive, etc.).

Even if no formal decision tree is constructed, clinical decision-making usually takes place along the lines of a decision tree. However, performing a formal decision analysis may be helpful in exactly defining each of the potential outcomes, pointing out the relevant (literature) data needed to make the analysis and estimating the utility of each of these potential outcomes. Furthermore, a decision tree may demonstrate the consequences of treatment when the diagnosis is uncertain or the treatment is sometimes unsuccessful and/or associated with complications, thereby offering useful guidance in clinical practice.

Further reading

Ingelfinger JA, *et al. Biostatistics in clinical medicine.* 3rd Edition. McGraw-Hill, Inc, New York, 1994.

Kassirer JP, *et al.* The toss-up. *N Engl J Med* 1981; **305:** 1467.

Sacket DL, *et al. Clinical Epidemiology: A basic science for clinical medicine.* 2nd edition. Little, Brown and Company, Toronto, 1991.

Weinstein M, Fineberg H. *Clinical decision analysis.* Toronto, Saunders, 1980.

IMPROVING PROFESSIONAL PRACTICE

Roland M. Valori

Even when clear guidelines and standards of care exist there can be wide variation in clinical behaviour and health outcomes. Some of this can be attributed to natural variation and some to biological variation in different populations. For example, death rates from coronary artery disease in hospitals serving populations at high risk might be expected to be higher (*BMJ* 2001; **322:** 184–185).

Variations in professional practice

However, some variation can be attributed solely to differences in professional practice. In extreme situations this behaviour might be regarded as negligent. More often there is either reduced quality of care or inefficient use of resource. In some circumstances, poor quality care will be cheaper. For example, failure to thrombolyse suitable patients presenting with myocardial infarction will save money, but the mortality rate for myocardial infarction will be higher.

In recent years there has been increasing awareness of variations in professional practice and with this, a desire to improve the practice of poorly performing doctors and other health professionals. This desire has led to increasing interest in the effectiveness of strategies to improve professional practice. Such strategies are amenable to experimentation in the same way as clinical questions on efficacy or causation. There is an expanding literature on the effectiveness of educational interventions aimed at improving professional practice.

Classic experimental study design is not the only evidence available to guide educators. There is a vast literature on adult education and change theory. Furthermore there is an emerging literature of qualitative and action research on changing professional practice. Readers who are interested in learning more about this area should read an excellent systematic review published in the Effective Health Care bulletin (*Effective Health Care* 1999; **5:** 1–15).

Experimental study designs

1. ***Randomized controlled trial.*** This is the gold standard study design for interventions aimed at improving professional practice. However, it is recognized that it is not always possible to conduct a randomized experiment, and two other study designs have achieved some respectability.

2. ***Controlled before and after study.*** This technique assesses the effects of an intervention by comparing change over time before and after an intervention, compared to change over an identical time period in a control group.

3. ***Interrupted time series.*** This study design assesses change after an intervention compared to a historical control period. There is no control group in this type of study.

The Cochrane Review Group on Effective Practice and Organisation of Care (EPOC) and the Heath Technology Assessment programme have published guidelines on the appraisal of these and other study designs (Cochrane Library 1998, *Health Technology Assessment* 1999; **3**(5)).

Appraisal

Whatever the type of study there are three components of educational interventions that deserve special attention: the population being studied; the intervention; and the outcome.

1. *Population.* The study population can be any group of health professionals, in any clinical setting. It is important to know details of the target population to determine whether the results are applicable in one's own setting. The majority of such studies have been done in North America and it is not clear how transferable the results are to Britain. For example the impact of a local opinion leader on 'office' physicians in the States may be quite different from that on British general practitioners.

2. *Intervention.* Unlike treatment trials, interventions aimed at improving professional practice usually have more than one component. For example, academic detailing delivered by a pharmacist or other health professional (what drug representatives do) may support guidelines in the form of printed materials. There is not a problem with multiple interventions; it just becomes difficult to determine which component of the intervention is more effective, or how dependent each one is on the others for its effectiveness. Furthermore it becomes very difficult to combine studies in the form of meta-analysis to give summary evidence of the effectiveness of interventions.

3. *Outcome measure.* Perhaps the most difficult aspect of these studies is the outcome measure. Ideally a study should use patient outcomes that the intervention is intending to modify through a change in clinical behaviour. For example, an educational intervention aimed at improving prophylaxis for deep venous thrombosis in patients undergoing hip replacement should use deep venous thrombosis, or pulmonary embolus, as the primary endpoint. In practice this would become a very complicated study to do, and it is likely that a surrogate outcome such as a measure of adherence to guidelines would be used in preference. The majority of published studies use health professional, or process outcomes, not clinical ones. Even when clinical ones are used, they are often surrogates for the outcome that really matters to the patient, e.g. blood pressure control rather than stroke.

Example

In this study of guideline implementation (*BMJ* 1993; **306**: 1728–1731) a guideline for the primary care management of infertility was embedded within a management sheet. Participants were randomized to receive the guideline or use normal management. Eighty-two practices were involved with 100 patients referred to hospital in both intervention and control groups. Outcome was in terms of sexual history, examination and investigation prior to referral.

Compliance with the guidelines improved for all targeted activities: e.g. history concerning couples use of fertile period, 85 *vs.* 69%, $P < 0.01$; examination of female partner 68 *vs.* 52%, $P < 0.05$; day 21 progesterone 72 *vs.* 41%, $P < 0.001$.

The study took place in Scotland in standard general practices. The intervention consisted of a two-sided A4 sheet which was used as a proforma by the GP and then sent to the hospital in place of a letter. This methodology seems generalizable to other areas and the setting was appropriate to general practice. However, infertility is a relatively specialized area in which GPs might have little experience. A guideline in a specialist area may be used differently to one for a more common disorder such as hypertension or asthma. Furthermore, infertility is unusual in that two people are being seen and investigated at once. This method of implementation can therefore be seen to be applicable to infertility in general practice but not necessarily to other clinical areas.

Further reading

Davis DA, Thomson MA, Oxman AD, Haynes RB. Evidence of the effectiveness of CME. A review of 50 randomized controlled trials. *JAMA* 1992; **268:** 1111–1117.

Haines A, Jones R. Implementing findings of research. *BMJ* 1994; **308:** 1488–1492.

NHS Centre for Reviews and Dissemination. Implementing clinical practice guidelines. *Effective Health Care* 1994; **8:** 2–11.

NHS Centre for Reviews and Dissemination. Getting evidence into practice. *Effective Health Care* 1999; **5:** 1–15.

Related topics of interest

Audit (p. 133); Guidelines (p. 136).

EXPLAINING RISK TO PATIENTS

William S.M. Summerskill

Evidence-based medicine is patient-orientated medicine. The chapters of this book are of little value, unless the potential benefits are realized in patient outcomes. EBM can help providers understand the individual implications of interventions through ORs, NNTs and CIs. Good communication skills are required to translate this information into concepts that health care consumers or planners can use.

A statistician described his profession as 'people who ate beef, but did not buy lottery tickets.' However, for most people decisions are based on values, as Kant observed: 'We see things not as they are, but as we are.' In a society where non-statistical assumptions influence behaviour, how can health care workers convey concepts of risk?

Perceptions of risk

Attitudes to risk are subject to three types of bias, which collectively form a 'lay epidemiology' in which perceptions are influenced by individual beliefs rather than fact.

1. Availability bias. The likelihood of an outcome is influenced by how readily examples come to mind. Rare events given prominent media attention will be perceived as more common than they actually are.

2. Confirmation bias. New evidence is manipulated (interpreted) to support existing opinions. Doctors can behave in a similar fashion when trying to confirm or refute a diagnosis.

3. Optimistic bias. Degree of an individual's confidence that he/she will be 'lucky' or 'unlucky' (pessimistic bias). This reflects underlying risk-taking or risk-aversion behaviour.

Concepts

Physicians are more likely to change behaviour when multiple interventions are used; so are patients. Combinations of verbal, numerical and graphical examples of risk are more effective than individual strategies (*BMJ* 1999; **319:** 749–752).

Absolute risk, relative risk, and cumulative risk are each important, and should be explained. Doctors, patients and the media can have difficulty placing relative risk in the perspective of absolute risk. Patients find relative risk more meaningful, although it can overestimate the overall benefit of an intervention. Cumulative risk describes the contribution of multiple factors in predicting outcome. An example is the influence of blood pressure, smoking and diabetes mellitus on the likelihood of individuals developing coronary heart disease, as in the *Joint British Societies Coronary Risk Prediction Chart* (*Heart* 1998; **80:** Supplement 2). A 'ladder of risks' (Table 1) may help patients to place a risk in perspective.

Table 1. Risk of an event in 1 year (After Calman, *BMJ* 1996; **313:** 799–802. Reproduced with permission)

Degree	Risk range	Example	Risk
High	>1:100	Gastrointestinal side effects of antibiotics	1:10–1:12
Moderate	1:100–1:1000	Death from smoking 10 cigarettes per day	1:200
Low	1:1000–1:10000	Death from road traffic accident	1:8000
Very low	1:10000–1:100000	Death playing soccer	1:25000
Minimal	1:100000–1:1000000	Death from railway accident	1:500000
Negligible	<1:1000000	Death from lightning Winning UK lottery (per game)	1:10000000 1:14000000

Examples of risk presentation

The way in which risks are presented affects decision-making (*NEJM* 1982; **306:** 1259–1262). This study asked doctors, patients and statisticians to imagine that they had lung cancer and then choose between two treatments based on factual data. Treatments were more likely to be accepted when presented in terms of survival rather than mortality. Prejudices about surgery *vs.* radiotherapy resulted in a greater preference for surgery when it was labelled as such, rather than when the treatments were compared anonymously as A and B.

Relative risk provides a more dramatic illustration of the potential benefit (or harm) of an intervention, and hence is popular with the media and pharmaceutical salespeople. Primary prevention of coronary heart disease in the *WOSCOPS* trial showed that cholesterol reduction could decrease the relative risk of a heart attack by 31% (*NEJM* 1995; **333:** 1301–1307). The findings are less impressive when presented in the context of absolute risk, where the risk of *not* having a heart attack increased from 93.3% to 93.8% (*BMJ* 1998; **316:** 1956–1958).

Approach

Three rules guide the explanation of risk:

1. Know the evidence. Like patriotism, evidence can be the last refuge of scoundrels. Be satisfied that the evidence is the most recent, most accurate, and most appropriate for the patient or population. Ensure that it has undergone critical appraisal by yourself or an independent body such as *ACP Journal Club* or *The Cochrane Collaboration.*

2. Know the audience. The existing doctor–patient relationship will provide a background, but not a substitute for the evidence. Trust is an important foundation for the patient believing the evidence that a clinician presents. Previous citations of poor evidence can compromise trust, whereas a relationship based on an open discussion of medical facts can foster trust. Select these messages carefully and reinforce them, using non-verbal information if necessary. Patients may only remember 20% of what they have been told, but recall can be doubled with visual aids (*Journal of the Royal College of General Practitioners* 1981; **230:** 553–556).

3.   Know the limitations   of evidence, personal knowledge and audience comprehension. Data are likely to be incomplete, particularly when trying to extrapolate findings to complex individuals. One's knowledge of evolving evidence is likely to be incomplete, or even biased.

Language or conceptual barriers may hinder communication. Keep it simple and involve translators or other family members when appropriate. Pain and emotions can also influence perception and decisions, so be sensitive. Remember that clinicians tend to underestimate the risks of interventions.

Further reading

Bennett P, Calman K (eds). *Risk Communication and Public Health.* Oxford: Oxford University Press, 2000.
Calman KC. Cancer: science and society and the communication of risk. *BMJ* 1996; **313:** 799–802.
Skolbekkon J.-A. Communicating the risk achieved by cholesterol reducing drugs. *BMJ* 1998; **316:** 1956–1958.

Related topics of interest

LIMITATIONS OF EBM

Roland M. Valori

The concept of evidence-based medicine evolved from clinical epidemiology, a discipline that has existed for many years. However, when EBM 'arrived' it was heralded as something new and it is therefore not surprising that there was a great deal of cynicism about its place in medicine. The original supporters of EBM were evangelical in their approach and their evangelism fuelled further cynicism. Things have settled down now so that the opinion leaders of EBM have a more pragmatic expectation of what EBM is, and what it isn't (*BMJ* 1996; **312:** 71–72), and the cynics complain less loudly than they did.

In the early years of EBM, it was accepted wisdom that if a patient did not fit the entry criteria of a study then the results of the study could not be applied to that patient. The tone has changed to a more moderate 'is my patient so different from those in the trial that its results cannot help me make my treatment decision?' (*How to practice and teach EBM*. London, Churchill Livingstone, 1997). This more realistic approach sums up the position of EBM today: it does not have the answer to every clinical question, but it does provide us with valuable additional evidence to help us make decisions.

The evidence of evidence-based medicine is just one type of evidence that we apply. There are other sources and we '. . . apply a sliding scale of importance to evidence from different sources that depends on the specific illness and patient' (*Lancet* 1996; **348:** 941–943). The key to integrating EBM into clinical practice is having it easily available and understanding its limitations. EBM helps shape, rather than make, clinical decisions.

Different observers will identify different problems with EBM depending on the perspectives of the culture they have developed in. Here are some issues that we regard to be important.

> **1. EBM is experimental and does not fit this patient.**   The most important thing to remember is that EBM is largely based on experimental data that show us how groups of patients, not individuals, respond to an intervention. However, it is often possible to apply trial data to individual patients, even if the patient would not have fitted the entry criteria for the study.

> **2. EBM misses important patient experiences.**   The classic large treatment trials miss out on all sorts of experiences which patients have as a result of their treatment. Often the question the trial has addressed will not be of prime importance to the patient, nor to the doctor looking after him. For example, the primary outcome of cancer trials is usually survival. Quality of life instruments (often derived from what doctors think is important) are secondary outcome measures, even when they may be far more relevant to the patient.

> **3. EBM favours interventions that attract commercial sponsorship.**   EBM is good for common disorders and for those that require a treatment or intervention that has a commercial application. Performing major randomized controlled trials properly is expensive and non-commercial research funds are scarce. This means that there is more, and better, evidence for commercial interventions than for non-commercial ones. A trial of physiotherapy for backache, or community psychiatric nurse visits for manic depressives will never get the financial backing that drug trials

attract. The result of this is that EBM will always create a bias in favour of interventions that can be sponsored. Many potentially effective, and possibly cheaper interventions will not receive health service funding because the 'evidence is not good enough', since there was never enough money available to test the intervention properly.

4. EBM is not accessible. Evidence exists in many forms and in many places. Until recently there have been problems accessing evidence in the clinic and at the bedside. New technology will improve accessibility but there remains a significant challenge to make evidence easy to assimilate. The Cochrane Collaboration is slowly bringing order to secondary research but reports of primary research still exist in a myriad of forms that are confusing to practising clinicians (see future of EBM). Furthermore the poor indexing of clinical trials can make searching for evidence a lottery for those who are unfamiliar with searching technique.

5. EBM cannot answer some questions. There is little doubt that the randomized controlled trial (RCT) is unable to answer all clinical questions, particularly those associated with rare diseases. However, there is a sufficient variety of other EBM techniques to enable us to address most questions the RCT cannot answer. Ultimately we rely on the best available evidence (which may be just a case series) to inform our clinical decisions.

6. EBM has limited value for purchasers of health care. Because much of EBM has been driven by the agenda of health professionals (principally doctors), purchasers of health care have a biased evidence base with which to make decisions. In the light of the NHS plan, purchasers will have to adapt their interpretation of evidence in the same way as clinicians adapt evidence according to their experience. Until recently most evidence was based on efficacy with relatively little cost data and even less information on the quantitative aspects of health gain. To make sensible purchasing decisions purchasers will need more economic analysis and much more sophisticated methods of assessing health gain so that competing interventions can be compared more easily.

7. EBM is misinterpreted and misused. None of us is free of preconceived ideas about diagnostic tests, causes of disease and the benefits and risks of treatment. Furthermore, patients, managers, the pharmaceutical industry, politicians, purchasers of health care and health professionals in other clinical settings will all have different priorities for different interventions. EBM is not always an exact science and it is not surprising that different groups within the health service will put their own spin on the results of a study. The key is to recognize that this will happen and make your own judgement about the evidence.

8. EBM is biased. There is no question that EBM is biased. The art of critical appraisal is to detect bias, determine whether it is influencing the results and, if so, in what direction.

THE FUTURE OF EBM

Roland M. Valori

Despite its limitations there is little doubt that EBM has an exciting future. There is a powerful demand for new evidence and for ways of getting evidence into clinical practice in the most efficient way. We can expect EBM to grow and evolve into many different forms as it permeates the consciousness of health professionals and the population at large. Technology will drive this change at a phenomenal pace and transform the things we are taught and the way we practice. Here is just a taste of where we think EBM is going.

Types of research – will we see more of the same?

The randomized controlled trial has been the emperor of EBM and will remain the gold standard design to which others will aspire. However, randomized trials will become more difficult to perform (see below) and there are questions that cannot be answered with RCTs. Other study designs will flourish where the RCT fails, but they will not ultimately replace it.

Change will occur because certain types of study will become easier to perform. For example large databases of clinical information will make it easier for case–control studies to be performed. At the push of a button, we will be able to do complex logistic regression analysis of the relationships of clinical conditions to a multitude of risk factors. However, we will have to be conscious of the problems associated with multiple testing, and hypotheses derived from these studies will need to be tested in further studies.

Change will occur as a much broader church of health professionals and patients become familiar with the principles of EBM. Doctors have been educated in a paternalistic, science-based culture that has meant that the priorities of the research community (until recently dominated by doctors and scientists) have not always coincided with the priorities of patients. The more patient-centred cultures of other health professionals will have a profound effect on EBM and result in a growth of qualitative research and greater emphasis on patient-centred outcomes.

New *in vivo* research methods such as outcomes research (see below) and action research will be refined and flourish. They will benefit from application of the principles of qualitative research and a better understanding of bias in research. They will always be subject to more bias than randomized controlled trials but they will not suffer the sampling problems that limit applicability of *in vitro* methods of research. These new methods will be championed by the managers of the health service responsible for delivering change and maximizing health gain from limited resource.

Older methods of research will be given a new lease of life with new applications. For example, the principles of diagnostic tests will be applied to symptoms and signs of disease. In future, the traditional list of symptoms we expect with a given disease, will also have a list of likelihood ratios for each symptom. These likelihood ratios will help us arrive at a differential diagnosis more efficiently, by enabling us to adjust the post-test odds of a diagnosis after each sign or symptom is elicited. Doctors taught to make diagnoses on the basis of probabilities will be better placed to help patients understand the diagnostic process and discuss uncertainties about diagnosis with them (in terms of levels of risk). This will enable them to share responsibility with patients for their decisions about diagnostic tests.

Study design and execution

The biggest change we can expect in conventional study design (i.e. that of the randomized-controlled trial) lies in development of the research question. There will be much greater emphasis of the importance of determining whether a question should be answered with further primary or secondary research (systematic reviews and meta-analysis). Both primary and secondary research questions will become more patient-centred and will better reflect the needs of practising health professionals, rather than those of the research, pharmaceutical or political communities. Greater emphasis will be placed on the inclusion of ethnic and other minorities in the formulation and prioritization of research questions. There will be an expectation that all major trials should include an economic evaluation.

Ethics committees will be more interested in the justification for a study, and they will look more closely at the study design and the ability of the researchers to complete it. This is because inadequately justified, poorly designed and incomplete studies that waste public funds and patients' time, are almost as unethical as those which are harmful to patients.

Randomized treatment trials will become more difficult to perform because new treatments are likely to have only marginal benefits over established treatments. Thus very large trials will be required to be reasonably certain of showing a difference or proving that one does not exist. This effect will be balanced both by increased public understanding of the need for RCTs, and by greater willingness to participate in clinical trials. This culture is already evident in the cancer patient population.

Better outcomes

More patient-centred outcomes (driven by the research question) will be commonplace. There will be major development and increased use of quality of life measures in clinical trials. Likewise, economic evaluations will be more usual and sophisticated. A persistent need for rationing of health care resource will drive refinement of the QALY (the currency of health gain) to enable competing health care interventions to be compared more easily.

Publication of research

We can expect a revolution in the peer review and publication process. Conventional peer review will become a thing of the past. Journals (if they still exist in 10 years) will no longer rely on the amateurish goodwill and inherent (but largely unintentional) bias of their reviewers. They will increasingly employ more professional reviewers and involve the public in their decision-making process.

Expect to see publication in cyberspace, under the auspices of current journals, of original research that has not been subject to traditional peer review. Journals will increasingly rely on the appraisal skills of their readers to make judgements about publications. Invited comments from readers and the ripostes from authors will ultimately determine the value of the research.

The authors of original research will commission their own reviewers, in much the same way as a person selling a house might commission an independent survey to reassure the purchaser that the house is sound. For example, most readers, without the necessary appraisal skills, might welcome an independent review of the statistical or economic analysis of a trial. It is possible for such reviews to be subject to bias in much the same way a household survey might ignore important defects; however, an independent 'appraisal agency' is unlikely to risk a long-term reputation for short-term rewards gained from intentional bias.

Conventional journals will not disappear any more than books or newspapers will. However they are likely to contain more summary evidence and original research presented within a set format, so that readers can assess the essence of a report or publication, without having to grapple with a particular presentation style.

Information

Most of us quickly forget knowledge or facts that we do not use regularly. In future we shall move from a culture of acquiring knowledge and memorizing facts to an information-finding one. This new way will have information instantly accessible, wherever it is needed: i.e. in the clinic or on the ward. In one study an 'evidence cart', containing various sources of evidence, was taken on ward rounds (*JAMA* 1998; **280:** 1336–1338). This evidence cart was too bulky to get close to the bedside but was a forerunner of what we may expect. In future it will be replaced by a small laptop (or similar device) attached to a ward trolley. With wireless internet link such a device will provide instant access to databases such as Cochrane and Medline, and also to local practice guidelines and protocols.

To make this development a reality (and practical) requires a change in the way information is organized and made available to health professionals. Currently information is available in many different databases and presented in confusingly different forms. Here is a shopping list of things we need (feel free to add a few of your own):

- fewer databases;
- better indexing and tagging of controlled trials;
- tagging discredited evidence;
- links to full text of original research or complete reviews;
- voice-activated searching, supported by artificial intelligence;
- local guidelines adapted from centrally tested evidence;
- summary evidence and primary evidence presented in a uniform format.

The biggest revolution, and the hardest one for the medical profession to get to grips with, will be the education of the general public in the principles of EBM. Currently it is commonplace for patients to consult, armed with information downloaded from the Internet. In the future, patients will have access to the same information we have, and some will have sufficient appraisal skills to challenge our interpretation of the evidence. For example, patients already have access to the electronic version of the BMJ.

Dissemination and implementation

Dissemination in this context refers to the release of research information up to the point it is incorporated into clinical practice. Variability in the application of evidence that cannot be explained on the basis of biological variation, and differences in resource allocation, will become increasingly poorly tolerated. Ironing out these differences will depend on a ruthless system of dissemination of best evidence and guidelines that will not clutter the everyday routine of practising clinicians. How will this happen?

Publication without peer review will speed up dissemination immensely. Sometimes evidence is not released for commercial reasons. To ensure equity of care in an organization like the NHS it seems reasonable that minimum and maximum (rationing) standards of care should be dictated from the centre. Thus the National Institute for Clinical Excellence and the National Service Frameworks (or similar alternatives) will continue to exist. They will be responsible for assimilating evidence and making judgements on what treatments are worthwhile, what can be afforded and what standards we can reasonably be expected to achieve, given a certain amount of resource. However, for effective implementation of best evidence to occur, local strategies are likely to be the most effective.

Withholding evidence will not be allowed. Compulsory registration of all controlled trials prior to ethical committee approval will reduce the chance of not omitting important trial results in systematic reviews. Furthermore, it will become unethical for commercially sponsored research on patients to be withheld from future publication.

In the future we can expect an explosion of models of implementation of evidence into practice. Most of these will not have been subject to a randomized design. Making sense of this new evidence will be a challenge. It seems likely that this mostly experiential evidence will be linked to more systematically derived (but more artificial) evidence in much the same way as clinical experience links with evidence-based medicine. The net effect will be substantial shortening of the dissemination and implementation time, and much less variation in practice.

Outcomes research

Outcomes research explores the relationship of outcomes to clinical behaviour and resource. The aim is to identify patterns of, or changes in, behaviour that are linked with particular outcomes. The value of outcomes research will increase as methods of recording clinical behaviour, resource use and outcomes improve.

Clinical outcomes will inform local guidelines

There is potential for clinical outcomes to be used to determine whether research results are worth applying in the local setting. The principle here is 'if it ain't broke don't fix it'.

Most treatment trials provide a number needed to treat (NNT) to prevent an event occurring over a defined period. For example, treating 20 patients with uncomplicated atrial fibrillation (AF) with warfarin will, depending on the age of the patient, prevent one stroke/year. If the number of patients with untreated AF within a defined area is known, the NNT enables us to calculate how many strokes we can expect to prevent if all these patients are anticoagulated. This expected benefit can be compared to the observed rate of AF-related stroke in the same area. If the expected benefit is greater than the observed rate the applicability of the trial (at least to this group of patients not already treated) should be seriously questioned.

Thus, comparing observed to predicted outcomes can help us test the applicability of a study in the local area and determine how an intervention is incorporated into local guidelines. In exceptional circumstances an intervention may not be implemented if a major mismatch is detected (no fix required). However, for smaller mismatches a subset of the population most likely to respond will be identified for treatment. This will be done with a combination of epidemiological and pharmaco-genetic techniques.

Preventative treatments such as statins for heart disease, cytoprotection for non-steroidal anti-inflammatory drugs and anti-resorptive agents for osteoporosis are ideally suited for this type of analysis.

Learning about EBM

Evidence-based medicine will become part of the curriculum for health professionals and the general public. It is a curious state of affairs that the Royal College of General Practitioners has EBM within the syllabus of the membership examination but the Royal College of Physicians does not. Appraisal of EBM is likely to become a 'life skill' for the general public.

Will the term evidence-based medicine survive?

No, but the concept will.

Further reading

Altman DG. The scandal of poor medical research. We need less research, better research, and research done for the right reasons. *BMJ* 1994; **308:** 283–284.

Begg C, Cho M, Eastwood S, *et al.* Improving the quality of reporting of randomized controlled trials. The CONSORT statement. *JAMA* 1996; **276:** 637–639.

Chalmers I, Dickersin K, Chalmers TC. Getting to grips with Archie Cochrane's agenda. All randomized controlled trials should be registered and reported. *BMJ* 1992; **305:** 786–787.

Leung WC, Whitty P. Is evidence-based medicine neglected by Royal College examinations? A descriptive study of their syllabuses. *BMJ* 2000; **321:** 603–604.

INDEX

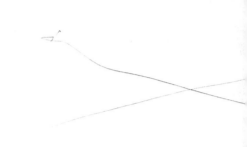